Interpersonal Skills f
People Professions

Learning from Practice

Interpersonal Skills for the People Professions

Learning from Practice

Edited by Lindsey Neville

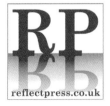

reflectpress.co.uk

First published in 2009

ISBN: 978 1 906052 18 8

British Library Cataloguing in Publication Data
A catalogue record for this book is available from the British Library

Production project management by Deer Park Productions
Typeset by Kestrel Data, Exeter, Devon
Cover design by Oxmed
Printed and bound in the UK by Bell & Bain Ltd, Glasgow

www.reflectpress.co.uk

Published by Reflect Press Ltd
11 Attwyll Avenue
Exeter
Devon, EX2 5HN
UK
01392 204400

Contents

List of Abbreviations

AL	Activities of Living
BACP	British Association of Counselling and Psychotherapy
BASW	British Association of Social Work
BM	blood sugar monitoring
BMA	British Medical Association
CAF	Common Assessment Framework
CBT	cognitive behavioural therapy
CEBSS	Centre for Evidence-based Social Services
CID	Criminal Investigation Department
CISD	critical incident stress debrief
CMC	General Medical Council
CPD	continuing professional development
CPR	cardio pulmonary resuscitation
CPN	community psychiatric nurse
CT	computerised tomography
CXR	chest X-ray
DCSF	Department for Children, Schools and Families
DDA	Disability Discrimination Act
DFES	Department for Education and Science
DNA	deoxyribonucleic acid
DOH	Department of Health
ECG	electrocardiogram
FBC	full blood count
FLO	family liaison officer
GCS	Glasgow coma score
GP	general practitioner
GSCC	General Social Care Council
GTC	General Teaching Council
HB	haemoglobin
HEI	higher education institution
HIV	human immunodeficiency virus
HMIC	Her Majesty's Inspectorate of Constabulary
ICM	International Confederation of Midwives
ICU	intensive care unit

INSET	in-service training
IS	information systems (previously information technology (IT))
ITU	intensive therapy unit (previously called intensive care unit)
MDT	multidisciplinary team
MIM	Murder Investigation Manual
MRI	magnetic resonance imaging
MS	multiple sclerosis
NAPWA	National Association of Police Welfare Advisers
NBM	nil by mouth
NGT	nasogastric tube
NUT	National Union of Teachers
NCALT	National Centre for Applied Learning Technologies – part of the distribution of learning programmes developed by NPIA
NICE	National Institute for Health and Clinical Excellence
NMC	Nursing Midwifery Council
NPIA	National Policing Improvement Agency
OIC	officer in charge – the police officer who conducts the main enquiries of an investigation
OT	occupational therapist
PACE	Police and Criminal Evidence Act 1984
PCSO	police community support officer – uniformed patrol staff with some powers to deal with offences
PDR	performance development review
PEACE	P = Preparation and planning
	E = Engage and explain
	A = Account
	C = Closure
	E = Evaluate
PIN	personal identification number
RDIM	Road Deaths Investigation Manual
RCPsych	Royal College of Psychiatrists
RTC	road traffic collision (often known as an accident)
SANDS	Stillbirth and Neonatal Death Society
SCIE	Social Care Institute for Excellence
SIO	senior investigating officer
SMARTER	action planning principle:
	S = Specific
	M = Measurable
	A = Achievable
	R = Realistic
	T = Time specific
	E = Evaluated
	R = Reviewed
SOCO	scene of crime officer

SOM	supervisor of midwives
TA	transactional analysis
TDA	Training and Development Agency
TSN	Teacher Support Network
WHO	World Health Organisation

Introduction

Lindsey Neville

ABOUT THIS BOOK

The inspiration for this book was the range of practitioners that I have been fortunate to work with in my professional life as both a teacher and a counsellor. I qualified as a teacher when I left school but, after many years of teaching in both primary and secondary schools, I realised that I was most interested in the pastoral side of work. Teaching and **counselling** are very different professions but do have one significant similarity in that to both teach and counsel you need to have an understanding of the difficulties faced by those with whom you work, and the ability to communicate that understanding. Increasingly, those people

> troubled by emotional difficulties tend to talk to whoever is at hand in their life who seems reliable and competent. A great deal of counselling, therefore, takes place in brief episodes, fitted into consultations with a doctor or nurse, or in the middle of a tutorial with a teacher, or in a conversation with a minister or priest. (McLeod, 2008)

McLeod goes on to describe this as an 'embedded role'. The counselling is set within another professional role. This embeddedness is clearly evident in the practice of the people professionals presented in this book.

I have chosen representatives from a number of different professions; however, I am also aware that many other people can provide effective support. For example, as a young student in the 1970s, my friends and I gained enormously from the listening ear of the cleaner who did our rooms in the halls of residence. She shared our joys and our woes, and sometimes just the telling was enough to change our day for the better. Many of us were away from our homes, families and life-long friends for the first time and, looking back, I think that her most valuable skill was making us feel that we mattered by giving us her time and a listening ear.

I am sure that there are times in your life when you have felt vulnerable, frightened or alone and a friendly word could make a difference. In my current work, as a Senior Lecturer in Counselling Psychology at the University of Gloucestershire, I am aware that, despite my responsibilities as a source of pastoral support for students, I may not be the person who is around when a student needs someone to talk things through with. It may be the security staff, porters, administrative, accommodation or catering staff who listen instead.

As a British Association of Counselling and Psychotherapy (BACP) Accredited Counsellor I contribute expertise in communication and **counselling skills** to a number of modules. In recent years I have been able to use an excellent range of different texts that support student learning in the development of basic communication and counselling skills. However, I have, for some time, been aware that there was little available that would support students in the way in which they might use these skills to support their service users. Consequently, this book is an attempt to fill that gap and allow students to understand how different practitioners apply theory to practice. I hope that the practitioners will also serve as role models and encourage you to consider a career in one of the people professions.

The people professions

Each chapter is written by a professional from one of the people professions:

- teacher;
- police officer;
- welfare officer;
- social worker;
- mental health nurse;
- nurse;
- midwife;
- general practitioner (GP).

By people professionals I mean all those who are committed to high standards in their work with people and, for most, this will also mean that they hold a professional qualification. They are professionals who are primarily seen for their main role but who need to use effective interpersonal skills to maximise their effectiveness. Each of the contributors has been selected for not only their background as a practitioner but also for their own excellent communication skills. It has not been possible to include representatives from all possible occupational settings – to have done so would have necessitated several volumes of this book! I am particularly aware that the ambulance service, physiotherapists, occupational therapists, audiologists, the prison service, the voluntary sector, alternative therapy practitioners and faith group leaders are not represented.

The background, age and gender of the professional will of course impact on their work. Men and women can bring different skills to the workplace and there is some evidence that in medicine, for example, women engage in more patient-centred communication (Roter *et al.*, 2002). It is for this reason that the contributors come from a variety of backgrounds, they vary in age from 32 to 63 and both men and women are represented.

The decision to use practitioners from a range of people professions rather than just those within health and social care settings reflects the need for professionals to work together in partnership. I hope that it will contribute to a greater understanding of the practice of others.

The values held by people professionals are central to their practice. These values will be developed as a result of the personal and professional belief system of each individual. Cuthbert and Quallington (2008) explore this core element of practice in more depth (further details can be found in the further reading section). Although this text is aimed specifically at health and social care practitioners, those involved in other areas of the people professions will find much of the discussion both interesting and helpful.

The structure of the book

The aim of the book is to present a variety of different ways in which effective interpersonal skills can be used. The practitioners will model a number of different ways of working with people using their greatest resource – themselves. They will explore issues that are central to their work and, with the help of case studies, present further discussion of:

- ethics and confidentiality;
- care of self;
- continuing professional development (CPD);
- training;
- boundaries;
- working with both service users and colleagues;
- the legislative context of their work;
- partnership working;

- practice skills;
- evidence-based practice.

Each chapter will begin with an editor's introduction, which seeks to identify common themes, and a pre-reading **reflection** activity, which will help you to begin to think about the issues that will be discussed.

You will quickly begin to see differences and similarities in the way in which each author uses communication and interpersonal skills. For example, as a counsellor I would rarely use closed questions with a client, believing that they limit and direct the response. Open questions put the client in charge of how much information they give. Similarly, Mary's welfare work (Chapter 4) in a large organisation relies on her ability to help her clients tell their story, which is more easily achieved with the use of open questions. On the other hand Lisa, as a nurse (Chapter 7), finds that closed questions enable her to elicit useful and necessary information. In the police service much of David's work (Chapter 3) necessitates the need to work with fact, for which closed questions are likely to be more successful. As you work through the book you will become aware of more examples of these similarities and differences. I hope you will also develop an understanding of the importance of professional collaboration, despite the tensions between professionals that are evident throughout the work.

Each chapter will conclude with key learning points, suggestions for further reading and reflection activities. A glossary is presented at the end of the text to provide a generic definition of the terms used in the book. However, throughout the book individual practitioners occasionally clarify their understanding and use of a particular term. Words included in the glossary are highlighted in bold in the text.

KEY THEMES

Service user perspective

The first chapter in this book takes the form of a discussion with Mike, a service user, and I am grateful to Mike for agreeing to be so honest about his feelings and experiences. His story highlights many of the issues that those of us who work with people need to address. We need to be ever mindful that we are visitors in someone's life and that we are there by invitation only. Service user needs should be at the core of our practice as people professionals. It is easy to become embroiled in the minutiae of our own professional concerns and to forget that, without the service users, we would have no profession to practise. I have used the term 'service user' to embrace the variety of terms used by different practitioners such as patient and client. Despite the current popularity of 'service user' the Royal College of Psychiatrists (RCPsych) (2003) found that in community health settings the use of 'patient' was preferred. You can read more about the different terms used for service users in Lindon and Lindon (2000).

Applying theory to practice

When I am working with students I know that they find it hard to equate theory with practice and yet it is central to the work of a people professional. Each of the people professionals in this text will discuss the theoretical models that underpin their individual practice. Inevitably there will be both similarities and differences as they discuss those models most applicable to the type of work that they do and those that are most appropriate to their own philosophy. Without exception each practitioner uses theory to inform their work. A range of theories is presented and you will be able to see how different professions make use of the same theory. The models presented include:

- Gerard Egan's 3 stage model;
- Carl Rogers' core conditions;
- Maslow's hierarchy of needs;
- Peplau's model of psychodynamic nursing;
- Roper, Logan and Tierney's model of nursing care;
- Betari's box;
- transactional analysis;
- Heron's intervention categories;
- Seden's model of surface and depth communication;
- Thompson's anti-oppression model;
- strengths perspective (Reynolds).

The use of case studies will enable you to see how people professionals apply theory to their practice.

Interpersonal skills

Interpersonal skills are needed to form and sustain helping relationships. They are all about working with people – people interacting with people. They include being able to support and encourage others, and being able to give and receive constructive criticism. They are also concerned with listening to and valuing others' thoughts and feelings. They are the skills that enable us to interact effectively with those around us. For the purposes of this text interpersonal skills are also viewed as a generic term that embraces a range of communication and counselling skills. These skills should be familiar to students who have embarked on a course leading to a qualification in the people professions. Those reading this who have not already gained some understanding and experience of these skills may find it helpful to read one of the texts recommended in the suggested further reading at the end of this chapter. The key skills used by the practitioners in this book include:

- reflecting;
- **paraphrasing;**
- **summarising;**
- questioning;
- **immediacy.**

Helping relationships

My practice has led me to conclude that there are two key elements essential to a helping relationship:

- being valued (we can demonstrate this by listening and giving time);
- being understood (we can demonstrate this by reflecting, paraphrasing and summarising).

Rogers (1959) identified three components for a successful helping relationship: **empathy, congruence** and **unconditional positive regard**. My experience in teaching counselling skills to students has been that they struggle with the language of the Rogers model and that at a base level students will embrace and act on a simpler model, that of valuing and understanding. This is not to imply that the Rogers model is unhelpful but that it is perhaps more usefully adopted at a later stage in training. A sympathetic approach has been scorned in recent years in favour of the Rogerian idea of empathy. It has been interpreted as 'feeling sorry' for someone. The Cambridge Dictionary (2008) actually defines sympathy as understanding and caring about someone else's suffering. It seems to me that this is an entirely appropriate approach towards service users by those in the people professions. If we don't care about other people's suffering perhaps we are in the wrong line of work. This concept of care is at the core of all of our work with people. Pickard (2000) highlights feedback from offenders who felt that the most noteworthy help that they had received from prison officers was that of care. Neville (2007) similarly highlights the importance of care for those in higher education. This includes our colleagues and partners as well as service users.

There is evidence that communication with health care professionals is a major cause of dissatisfaction and that good communication has a positive impact on health (Roberts *et al.*, 2001). It can be the simplest of skills that will encourage someone to tell you their story. Author and lecturer Leo Buscaglia once talked about a contest he was asked to judge. The purpose of the contest was to find the most caring child. The winner was a four-year-old child whose nextdoor neighbour was an elderly gentleman who had recently lost his wife. Upon seeing the man cry, the little boy went into the old gentleman's garden and just sat there beside him. When his mother asked what he had said to the neighbour, the little boy said, 'Nothing, I just helped him cry' (Canfield and Hansen, 1996).

It is particularly important for readers to be clear about the differences between using a range of what are now widely called counselling skills and the practice of counselling. Donnelly and Neville (2008) discuss the differences between the two and provide activities to support students who are developing their interpersonal skills.

As people professionals it is almost inevitable that we will meet people when they feel at their lowest and therefore their most vulnerable. This might be for any one of a number of reasons including:

- a bereavement;
- an illness;
- making a difficult decision;
- a difficult life event.

This increases the sense of responsibility that I feel for my clients' well-being. In my own professional life as a counsellor I am acutely aware that no one comes to see me to share their joy. As they tell me their story clients also confide in me their experiences of other professionals that they meet on their journey and I am sometimes shocked by the stories that they tell. I recently had my own experience of an outpatient's clinic in which:

- the consultant did not introduce himself;
- the consultation was conducted with the door open so that my personal information was relayed to those sitting in the waiting area outside the room;
- throughout the consultation he called me Lesley (despite the fact that my name is Lindsey!).

When the consultation was over I was left feeling of very little importance.

In our busy working lives it is easy to forget the impact of our actions (albeit sometimes unintentional). Given that mental health problems are the largest single cause of disability and illness in England, accounting for 40 per cent of all physical and mental disability and a third of all GPs' time (Department of Health (DoH), 2008), it is likely that a large proportion of those whom we will meet professionally may also be struggling to deal with a mental health illness, increasing their vulnerability.

Recognising our own limitations

There is a debate about whether **counselling skills** training should be a normal and necessary part of the training for all those who assist others to manage problem situations. However, Stokes (2001) argues that 'training is not always necessary to help people' (p. 133) but an understanding of boundaries and ethical issues may be beneficial. If professionals learn to recognise their own limitations then they will be able to develop an awareness of the situation when they may be out of their depth. This feeling of being out of one's depth occurs when the needs of the service user exceed the practitioner's knowledge and experience. Having recognised your own limitations means it will be necessary to be able to identify more suitable sources of help and support so that the service user can be referred appropriately.

Evidence-based practice

Inevitably people professionals will come from very different backgrounds with different sets of personal values. Additionally, each professional setting will have its own set of values. Evidence-based practice will ensure that 'decisions about health care are based on the best available, current, valid and relevant evidence' (Dawes *et al.*, 2005) rather than being based solely on these individual or contextual values.

The Centre for Evidence-Based Social Services (CEBSS, 2004) highlights a number of ways in which practitioners might ensure that their practice is evidence-based. These include:

- journal groups;
- team meetings;
- newsletters;
- circulating research;
- forming links with university departments.

As you read through the chapters you will be able to identify different ways in which each professional ensures that their practice is evidence-based.

IN CONCLUSION

As you read this book I hope that you will begin to define and describe what it really means to care and to develop a range of ways in which you can develop the skills you will need in the workplace. Personally I feel that there can be no more rewarding and challenging work than helping individuals to develop and adjust to the circumstances in which they find themselves. I hope that you will find that the same is true for you.

REFLECTION ACTIVITIES

1. Effective interpersonal skills are not exclusively the domain of those working in the field of health and social care. Try to think of other workers who may use interpersonal skills to help or support their service users.
2. Think about a time when you have listened to someone else's problems. What difference did it make to both you and them?

FURTHER READING

Cuthbert, S. and Quallington, J. (2008) *Values for Care Practice*. Exeter: Reflect Press

Donnelly, E. and Neville, L. (2008) *Communication and Interpersonal Skills*. Exeter: Reflect Press

Geldard, D. and Geldard, K. (2005) *Counselling Skills in Everyday Life*. Basingstoke: Palgrave

Lindon, J. and Lindon, L. (2000) *Mastering Counselling Skills*. Basingstoke: Palgrave

Chapter 1

The Service User Perspective

Mike Alan and Lindsey Neville

EDITOR'S INTRODUCTION

In this chapter you will read a conversation between Mike Alan, a service user, and Lindsey Neville, a BACP accredited counsellor and senior lecturer in Counselling Psychology at the University of Gloucestershire. It is presented at the beginning of the book to highlight that the work that we do with clients, patients and service users affects their lives. I would go even further and remind the reader that through some periods of extensive treatment or professional involvement it might actually be their life. Their experience of us as professionals can have a profound effect on their experience of their disability/illness and their ability to cope with difficult and challenging circumstances. It is also about acknowledging that service users have work responsibilities, parents, partners, children and social lives.

In 2001 Mike was diagnosed with multiple sclerosis (MS). Multiple sclerosis is the most common, disabling neurological condition in the UK, affecting approximately 85 000 people. It is the result of damage to the protective sheath that surrounds the nerve fibres of the central nervous system. This interferes with messages between the brain and other parts of the body. MS is sometimes characterised by periods of relapse and remission, while for others it has a progressive pattern (MS Society, 2007). Once present the disease never goes; there is no cure and the person lives with the diagnosis for life (National Institute for Health and Clinical Excellence (NICE), 2003).

Mike's discussion of his experiences of the interpersonal skills of the professionals that he has met in the lead up to and since his diagnosis highlight what I have observed in my professional life regarding the forgiving nature of many service users. Mike's words enable us to see what works and what doesn't work for him but it is important to remember that people have differing needs and that what works for one won't necessarily work for others. For example, on page 15 he talks about what I perceive as the poor interpersonal skills of the neurological consultant. Mike, however, grew to like and respect him for his 'straight talking'.

Key themes

- Service user perspective.
- Diversity.

Pre-reading reflection activity

In this chapter Mike talks about an almost throwaway remark by one of his teachers in which he was told that he would never make an officer in the Marines. You will see that he was driven to prove the teacher wrong, which defined his future. Think about the power of such remarks and reflect on the impact of any that you might have received yourself.

MIKE ALAN – SERVICE USER

Lindsey: Tell me a little about yourself

Mike: I was born into a services family and spent the first ten years of my life travelling before being sent off for a settled secondary education at an all male naval boarding school. I was younger than the majority of my academic year which left me a little insecure and with a need to compete to prove myself. I enjoyed sport, particularly rugby, and represented the school rugby, tennis and athletics teams, eventually winning the Suffolk AAA youth shot put competition. I was a strong swimmer, gaining a life-saving distinction award and a mile swim certificate. It is fair to say that, despite carrying a little too much around my midriff, I have always enjoyed good health and outdoor activities.

While studying for my 'A' levels, I was determined that I would join the Royal Marines. I remember as I set off for an initial interview in Admiralty House, my house master called me to one side and said, 'I don't know why you are wasting their time; you will never make an officer'. Two years later, he did the same to my brother who wanted to try for an Army commission. My brother was put off by the comments and carved out a different career. I was fortunate enough to be accepted into the Corps and served a five-year short-service commission. (In Chapter 2 Wendy explores the use and importance of interpersonal skills in education.)

Having left the Royal Marines I eventually served as a police officer for 24 years. Throughout my service I never worked for more than two years in any one position so I gained wide experience, having worked the beat in cities, towns and villages and spending time out of uniform as a detective.

Lindsey: **Your working life has brought you into contact with a wide range of different people. You must have gained an insight into what people find helpful when they are in a crisis.**

Mike: The roles I undertook meant dealing first-hand with the public at their most vulnerable and disempowered: whether they were victims of crime, recovering from involvement in a road traffic collision, being told that a close relative had just died or frustrated at being arrested, the emotions are varied and the biggest lesson I learned was that reactions could not be predicted. As my career progressed, I was involved in training, personnel, operations, custody centres and the internal inspection process. All these roles involved challenging the way people managed their lives and often meant having to deal with them feeling defensive. Again, reactions of even the most professional individual could not be predicted. I learnt to remember that one never knows the circumstances that people are already dealing with at the time when we meet with them. Some of my roles involved working in a multi-agency environment where stereotyping on all sides often resulted in time having to be spent building trust before real progress could be made.

Lindsey: **It sounds as if you led a very active life, working with different groups of people. You have told me that throughout your working life, despite your high levels of fitness, you found physical exercise inexplicably fatiguing. How did you address the concerns that were growing about your health?**

Mike: Yes, it was an active life, so I became quite concerned around 1992 when, during a game of squash, I found I could not see any ball being hit down the right-hand side of the court; it was as though someone had smeared Vaseline across my eye. Yet, when tested, I was able to see quite normally. I went to my GP who could not diagnose a problem and referred me to an ophthalmic specialist; he appeared dismissive of any problem and said that if I was worried I should just see a high-street optician. The optician could find no impairment and suggested it might be optical migraine. This whole series of visits was concerning because I knew there was something wrong and therefore could not understand why no one was giving me a diagnosis – it was as though I was being called a liar. However, my system seemed to agree with the specialists because six months later I was back to normal, as suddenly as it had started. What was frustrating about all these professionals was that, once they told me they had no diagnosis or explanation to offer, I was left in limbo, 'Well, you could always try . . .' and so it was left to me to make my own enquiries and chase up leads. It felt as if there was no continuity of care.

Lindsey: So it sounds like no one accepted any responsibility for helping you to find a diagnosis, you felt 'passed around'?

Mike: Yes and things continued to deteriorate. Some four years later I developed numbness and tingling in various parts of my lower limbs after I had walked for 15 minutes or so. I lived with this for a couple of years without complaining, putting it down to sciatica then, one day, while crossing a road in a town centre, I found myself flat on my face for no reason that I could fathom; my momentum had kept going but my left leg had simply stopped working. Again, my GP had no explanation for what might be wrong, nor did he refer me to anyone else. The numbness started to spread and become more defined around my crotch area after about 15 minutes walking. In late 2000, I sought the services of a sports physiotherapist and finally found someone who seemed to take a real interest, asking extensive questions about symptoms I had experienced and really listening to my answers. He made me exercise so that I could experience the sensation during his examination. He wrote a comprehensive report which I was able to take to a doctor; I saw him socially some time later, after my diagnosis, and he said 'I suspected as much, but it was not my place to tell you.' I can appreciate that he did not want to worry me with a false diagnosis but I was worrying anyway, which was the reason I had visited him.

By now I had moved house and, on changing my GP, I told him that if I was a car, I would be asking for a major overhaul as so many bits seemed to be going wrong with me. He took the physiotherapist's report and started to send me for a series of investigative tests. Despite me asking what he was testing for, he wouldn't tell me, just saying it was preferable to eliminate all possibilities rather than draw conclusions. However, within a month or so, I was referred to a consultant neurologist. To speed the matter, I went privately. He too started a series of tests but without letting me know what his thought processes were. He told me he was making an appointment for me to have a magnetic resonance imaging (MRI) scan on both my back (the source of a great deal of my pain) and my brain. Now that gave me real cause for concern; as far as I was being told, there was nothing for me to worry about, yet I was about to be subjected to a machine which would examine all my inner workings.

In the event, I had to move house to a different county and transferred GP again, at the same time being referred to a National Health Service (NHS) neurologist. The MRI process was undertaken in September 2001 and I was told I would be given the results once they had been read by a specialist.

Lindsey: You had been through so much. How did you eventually get a diagnosis?

Mike: One day in early November, I had a phone call from my GP to say the neurologist wanted to see me as soon as possible and would I be able to attend a clinic in a town some twenty miles distant [not his usual surgery] a couple of days later. He went on to say, 'It might be an idea if you took your wife along or someone else who can drive you home.' No explanation, even when I pressed him . . . Was I worried? Oh yes! I fretted for days.

My wife and I went to the clinic and we were called in to see the consultant. We were last on the surgery list and had no idea what to expect. This doctor wasted no time when he saw us. He asked us to sit down and said 'I now have the results of your scan, you have multiple sclerosis and it is secondary progressive.' He said he was sure we would have a lot of questions but suggested we read some pamphlets which he gave us together with the contact details for the MS nurse and suggested we made an appointment to meet with her. He said he could understand if we were worried but that he would be unable to give the answers to the questions we were likely to have because the illness is so unpredictable. He pointed out that progression had been slow until that point but that he could still give no prediction. The one point he made that is still clear was that 'MS is not a terminal disease'.

Over time and a dozen consultations since, I have grown to respect and like the man although I am aware that many of his patients and working colleagues regard him as a cold fish, lacking in people skills. Certainly there was no warmth about him at that appointment, everything was a matter of fact, there were no smiles and no sympathy. We walked away to the car and I am not even sure that the suggestion that my wife drive home was a wise one. Both our minds were working overtime, we spoke about a multitude of things, whether I could continue to work, what we had both heard about the illness, what our financial position might be, whether I should try and take time off work, whether I would need a wheelchair and in consequence whether we would have to move out of our recently purchased house. We missed three turnings to our home town.

Before long, however, my response to the diagnosis was one of relief. I now had a hook I could hang things on and it offered an explanation for many of the health issues with which I had had to contend. Over time I was able to distinguish what were probably symptoms of MS and what were other health issues.

Lindsey: You were a senior police officer so what problems did the early stages of the illness cause in the workplace? Did other people help or hinder?

Mike: Immediately following my diagnosis, I was feeling knocked sideways. I didn't know what MS really was, how it would affect me, whether I was now life-limited, etc. I had been advised to see or contact a number of people: the MS nurse, the MS Society, my GP, a physiotherapist, an occupational therapist (OT) and so on. I had also been told that, for now, I could continue to work.

My father had died relatively young at 63 having left, until he was retired, all those big holidays and hobbies to pursue. I didn't want to feel that I was left with regrets that I had not achieved. However, I didn't know if I could afford to give up work to go and do them. So I therefore also needed to find out what pension I could get and whether I could afford to leave my job. I was in such mental turmoil, I wanted all this to be organised straight away.

At the time, my department was going through a major review and I had my finger very much on the pulse – more so than my line manager. Because of the workload, he had banned all annual leave and I didn't feel it would be morally right to 'pull a sicky'. I wasn't sick, I had an illness! I went to see him and said 'I need some time off, I would rather not give you a reason, please just trust me that it's necessary and I would not ask if it wasn't, I only need a couple of days' (I already had people lined up to see). He replied 'Not good enough, I will need to have a reason.' So I said 'OK, I will tell you, but I want you to keep it strictly confidential.' I told him and his response was 'I can't let you have the time off, you know how busy we are, what am I supposed to do? Oh, and I will have to tell the Chief Constable, I can't keep that to myself.' I lost it – I felt totally disempowered. After a while I worked out for myself how he could cover me if I did go off and I was allowed to do so. He told me he would respect my wish for confidentiality.

Compare that with a few days later when I had seen the people I needed to see and made my decision to take early retirement. I phoned the Chief's office and asked if I could have five minutes of his time for personal reasons. I was told he could squeeze me in briefly between two senior officers if I felt it was genuinely important. I arrived at his office, he invited me in and asked what the problem was. I said 'I have come to ask if I can retire on ill health grounds.' He immediately ordered coffee for us both and asked how he and the Force could help me; he went on to give me half an hour of his time, making other people wait while he talked through various welfare issues. What a difference . . .

Lindsey: How have you coped/managed things?

Mike: We got home and spent hours in front of the computer trying to find out what we could about the disease. As I have said, in many ways, my initial reaction to the diagnosis was one of relief. I was still frightened. I had visions of wheelchairs and there were too many articles available about the illness causing the break up of people's marriages or the loss of friends, or having to be peg-fed [a tube into the stomach].

In the event, I retired from the police service. I tried to draw up a list of the things I wanted to do in life, which turned into a list of places I wanted to see. I went to a travel agent and gave a young trainee my list, explaining my predicament and that one day I might be faced with being a wheelchair user. She immediately grasped the issue and asked me to take a seat while she listened to how I might need assistance and what I wanted from each place and then asked me to give her some time to research my list. Within a couple of days she had phoned me back with my list prioritised as requested and her good wishes in achieving my goal. She made no effort to impose on me by trying to sell me my first holiday and the way that she responded to me probably led to an upturn in the way I started to view my life. I think that the reason for this was that she was young and naive and, I think, taken aback at the task I had set her – and it was actually her lack of skill which helped. She didn't treat me as different – it was almost that way that youth has of taking things in their stride; she just regarded it as a challenge to help someone who had presented her with a task. She was not at all patronising but she came across as being interested in me as a person and took the problems I might face as a matter of fact, rather than viewing me as an illness.

Retirement did not last long, just six months while I tried filling my time by starting a number of hobbies – woodturning, painting and playing a musical instrument – but actually found I missed working so I volunteered as a tutor on the NHS Expert Patient Programme, became active in the local and regional branches of the MS Society and eventually took employment again as a mentor for the disabled service users of Leonard Cheshire Disability. I am one of a national team of 20 disabled people and, looking back, I am able to see how my attitude towards coping with my own illness has changed. Initially my colleagues would tell me I had 'not embraced the fact that I was a disabled person'. I could not see it until one day it was pointed out at a staff meeting that I was still referring to disabled people as 'them'. I realise now that I was probably judging myself by the visible impairments that are the standards by which disability is normally judged and, while I was still able to walk around and speak normally, in my own mind I was not really disabled even though the Disability Discrimination Act (DDA) had defined me disabled from the point of my diagnosis.

When I am asked how having the illness has affected my life I joke that I don't suffer from MS but am making a living from being a disabled person. Apart from my role of mentor, I train in disability equality, I undertake disabled accessibility audits and I give talks to police officers on how disability can impact on people's lives. My job takes me to venues across the South West and I find that driving can be very tiring, especially if I have had to concentrate hard at work throughout the day. Fortunately the government has a scheme known as 'Access to Work' that is available to help overcome the problems resulting from disability. It offers practical help in a flexible way which, for me, means having the services of a driver to take me to and from places of work.

My mobility gives problems in a number of ways – sometimes I stagger through fatigue, other times I lose balance. I have had a mixture of symptoms from dropped foot, to being unaware of where my limbs are spatially. This caused me confusion over whether I should use sticks, crutches or just stagger, until one day my wife took me shopping and I used a shopping trolley. Suddenly I found I was able to walk normally without a limp, a stagger or a swerve. I decided to be assessed to see whether a walking frame with wheels might be beneficial. A private occupational therapist discussed with me the benefits of which one to use and I went to social services to ask them if they would provide one.

I was told they couldn't as they only provided equipment for use inside the home so, if I needed equipment for external use, I would have to seek help from the NHS. I talked the problem through with my designated NHS physiotherapist who agreed a frame would be ideal for me but who told me she was unable to help as equipment was only available for people coming out of hospital on rehabilitation. I ended up buying my own frame. On its first outing, I visited an antiques fair. I was followed by an older couple who my wife heard having a conversation about me. Him: 'Why is that man taking up so much room with that walking frame, he obviously doesn't need it?' Her: 'He must be a mental case then.' I have not used the frame since.

My house was a split-level design with the main living accommodation on the first floor. About a year after diagnosis, I was finding great difficulty negotiating the stairs so we looked for a bungalow. Not knowing what the future had in store but anticipating the possibility of a wheelchair, I decided that as the new home needed work to be done anyway, it would be as well to have things prepared for the 'just in case'. Ramps were built to the front and rear doors, wider doors were put in the main entrances and in the rooms I would have to use and a wheelchair-accessible bathroom was installed.

Lindsey: Since diagnosis, what have been your experiences of the range of people involved in ensuring you get the best possible treatment and care?

Mike: For some years now, the MS Society has funded specialist nurses in various regions nationally. In November 2003, the NICE produced guidelines for the management of MS in primary and secondary care (NICE, 2003) and once 'in the system' I found it relatively easy to get referrals to a range of specialists. These included an MS specialist nurse, a neuro-physiotherapist, bladder control specialist nurse, bowel control specialist nurse, sexual dysfunction specialist nurse, radiologists and psychologists. I have been fortunate enough to be included on a beta-interferon programme and have had little difficulty obtaining steroid treatment when I have felt it would be beneficial. I know I have been lucky; both my GP and my consultant neurologist are understanding and happy to listen to me. Or, perhaps, I am fortunate enough to be able to communicate in an effective way (and having the ear of the neurologist's personal assistant has been helpful!). Recently I have been fortunate to work with an occupational therapist who has referred me to wheelchair services, shortcutting an extensive waiting list. Outside the health service, I have been able to obtain speedy appointments with the local social services, which has enabled me to get different equipment for the house.

I am aware that not everyone in my shoes has been able to access services with the relative ease I have found. However, accessing the services is of no great benefit if the service received falls short of acceptability.

Lindsey: What could any of the practitioners, who you have met throughout your illness, have done to make things better/clearer/easier for you?

Mike: Most commonly, the experience I have had has been that people have been so keen to impart information that I have sometimes come away from appointments wondering what has been discussed. I have learnt to write a list of questions before attending appointments, but am not always in a position to take notes during the course of an appointment. My questions are therefore addressed but, when I try to recall them later, the answers become a blur. I now ask the specialists to send me a copy of any letters written as a result of any consultation but this still does not necessarily cover all aspects raised.

There are a number of things that the professionals could do to help me cope with the debilitating effects of MS. The main symptom experienced by people with MS is fatigue, and so I like to plan my life as much as possible.

- It would be nice to be offered options for appointments – days of the week and times of the day. This would make symptom management easier.
- The offer of copies of file notes or even a written note to take away of salient points would be useful.
- Ensure that a directory of services is available so that when a referral is made all the information is to hand.
- Suggest that carers might want to attend – and watch for their needs and fears as well as the person who is the main recipient of your time.

Lindsey: How were your family and friends affected by your illness? How did it change how they communicated with you – or you with them?

Mike: My stock answer to this question used to be that family and friends have been very supportive. And, generally speaking, they are. Deeper and more honest analysis reveals a different picture in respect of their individual ability to cope.

- My mother will read no information about my illness in case it should reveal what she fears about how I might become. She reads news items about so-called 'miracle cures' and immediately wants to spend money on them for me, without wondering whether they really work.
- My best friend, despite being the first to contact me with the most wonderful letter of support, still cannot cope with seeing me struggle physically.
- Close neighbours and friends who had learned to cope with my almost perpetual limp went off into a fit of giggles when they saw my arm go into a spasm and raise itself into the air . . . Instead of laughing with me I felt that they were laughing at me which, in turn, embarrassed me.
- My wife has been very supportive and cares for me. However, our relationship has been very strained of late because I not only need someone who cares, but a carer who will help rather than insisting that I not undertake an activity. Some physical activities will reduce me to a weakened shell. For example, I still like to cut the grass, but I know that if I cut more than a certain amount of the lawn, I am likely to have to crawl back to the house (or maybe even just sit where I am on the grass for half an hour to recover). However, knowing the likely consequences, it is then my choice whether to get the lawn mower out of the shed and the last thing I want to hear is a demand for me not to start in the first place. I don't want to just sit in the sun and grow old and watch other people cut my grass – or, more likely, wait for someone to cut my grass and then do it badly!

Key learning points

- Service users have different expectations for, and needs from, the professionals that they come into contact with.
- Carers have needs too.
- Relationships with partners come under increased strain when one of the couple has a disability or illness.
- Service users need some continuity of care.
- Support can be found from unexpected sources.

REFLECTION ACTIVITIES

1. Try to put yourself in Mike's position. You are being told that you have a serious illness for which there is no cure. What expectation do you have of the person who is telling you the news? How might you go about telling the news to the people who love you?
2. Identify and evaluate the communication and interpersonal skills used by the professionals in Mike's story.

FURTHER READING

Barnes, C. and Mercer, G. (2006) *Independent Futures: Creating User-led Disability Services in a Disabling Society*. Bristol: Policy Press

Rose, D. (2001) *Users' Voices: The Perspectives of Mental Health Service Users on Community and Hospital Care*. Sainsbury's Centre for Mental Health

Chapter 2

Interpersonal Skills in Education

Wendy Messenger

EDITOR'S INTRODUCTION

In this chapter you will read about the work of a teacher in a primary school.

Research highlights that those with good social skills, including interpersonal skills, are most likely to do well for themselves in later life (Goleman,1996). In recent years this has become part of government education policy with all schools emphasising the importance of positive communication in developing social skills. Wendy highlights the challenges that these multi-layered interactions may pose as practitioners both teach and model positive interpersonal skills for their pupils.

Given the importance of safeguarding children it will be apparent that the question of ethics and confidentiality is central to the practice of a teacher. The dilemmas that this can create are explored and related to the significance of reflection and evidence-based practice.

Key themes

- Ethics and confidentiality.
- Diversity.
- Reflection.
- Evidence-based practice.

WENDY MESSENGER – PRIMARY SCHOOL TEACHER

Describe the kind of interactions that you might have with people in the course of a normal working day

A teacher is engaged in many different kinds of interactions during the school day that are often demanding and complex. As a primary school teacher, the following was a typical day:

- At 8.30 a.m. I attended a briefing meeting with staff colleagues to discuss significant issues for the day in school, including arrangements for timetabling, visitors to the school and staffing rotas.
- At 8.45 a.m. I rushed off to a planning meeting with the teaching assistant who works with me to share information and ideas for the teaching activities and resources required for that day.
- At 9.00 a.m. the children came into the classroom and my teaching started.
- At 10.30 a.m. it was my turn for playground duty, which involved supervising all the children in the school during their break, including organising first aid and sorting out disputes and arguments and disciplining pupils when appropriate.
- At 12.00 noon break for lunch finally arrived. I met with the educational psychologist for half an hour who was in school to discuss the progress of a child in my class and to review strategies that I had been using to support his learning.
- At 1.00 p.m. the children came back into the classroom for the afternoon and my teaching started again.
- At 3.30 p.m. I had a meeting with the parents of a child in my class who came to discuss how they could help their children more at home.
- At 4.30 p.m. I met with the head teacher to update her on the progress of the children deemed to be gifted and talented in my class.

A deeper analysis of these interactions that I was involved in during this day reveal a wide range of interpersonal communication at different levels. They would seem to be some of the ones Hayes (2002) suggests:

- awareness of self and others;
- listening;
- questioning;
- presenting information to others;
- helping and facilitating;
- asserting and influencing;
- negotiating.

It is interesting to note that as a teacher these skills are required at different levels to match the partner or partners in communication who may be pupils, colleagues, parents/carers or other professionals. Milner-Bolotin (2007) draws an analogy between teaching and acting; they both depend upon the interaction between the teacher (the actor) and the pupil/parent/colleague/other professional (audience). The teacher must be sensitive to the audience's ability to understand the communication and will need to consider maturation, attitude, emotional state and ability to understand. In the example above, during playground duty I was interacting with children who were at different ages and stages of their development so, in attempting to support them to resolve conflicts in the playground, my questioning, asserting, influencing and negotiating skills had to be responsive to this.

The environment in which the interactions take place is also important. In the example above, my meeting with the parents took place in a small comfortable meeting room that was private rather than the classroom or within the hearing of other parents or pupils.

What are the skills that you use in your work with people?

> I've come to the frightening conclusion that I am the decisive element in my classroom. It's the personal approach that creates the climate. It's my daily mood that makes the weather. As a teacher, I possess a tremendous power to make a child's life miserable or joyous. I can be a tool of torture or an instrument of inspiration. I can humiliate or humour, hurt or heal. In all situations, it is my response that decides whether a crisis will be escalated or de-escalated and a child humanised or de-humanised. (Ginott, 1972)

This quotation had a great impact on me as a young teacher and helped me to realise the enormity of my responsibility to my pupils.

Case study

Eight-year-old Adina, a relative newcomer to the school, was always a challenge in my maths lessons. She would attempt to disrupt in any way she could by calling out, complaining about her peers and refusing to do the tasks set. It was difficult to teach her, or to teach the others sometimes.

I decided to choose Adina to be classroom helper for the week, which involved her staying behind for a short time at break time to help organise and tidy the classroom resources. It provided an opportunity for her to tell me that she found maths difficult in her last school and got left further and further behind. As a result she was teased by her friends.

In the maths lessons the following week, I made some changes. I made sure she received stickers for participating in the lesson, that I set tasks that we agreed were achievable, but still had to be done, and praised her efforts and celebrated her achievements in front of her friends. Whenever there was a time when she started to interrupt the lesson, I gave her 'the look' and a private signal which involved me touching my head to indicate 'remember what we agreed'.

The skills I was using on this occasion were what Carl Rogers (1959) would term '**unconditional positive regard**'. They were varied and at times multilayered, but underpinning my strategies was my belief that positive relationships with children are the key to positive behaviour and children behave well when they feel valued and that they belong. This is a view also articulated by the Department for Education and Skills (DfES, 2005) in the Primary National Strategy. Hook and Vass (2000) propose that teaching requires you to enter the pupil's world in order to influence them and support them. I needed to demonstrate empathy and establish trust with Adina and sought to do this by trying to understand why she behaved in the way she did. I provided a context, a private space during break time, in which to establish this.

Non-verbal language is very powerful, including facial expression, tone and volume of voice, and gesture. I was able to use this to good effect by establishing a signal Adina and I understood that gave the message of my expectations and reminded her of what we agreed. We had negotiated between us what our expectations were of each other, which helped Adina to feel that I valued her and that I had taken her views into consideration. Use of positive motivation was also important and the celebration of Adina's achievements in front of her peers helped raise her self-esteem. 'Catching her being good' is a strategy I used, rather than one that would have been construed as bribery.

In 2000 the Department for Education and Employment (DfES) commissioned research into what Year 8 pupils thought were the qualities of a good teacher. While this is not the complete list, it is interesting to note that many of these are related to the 'interpersonal skills' of teachers.

A good teacher:

- listens to you;
- encourages you;
- takes time to explain things;
- helps you when you get stuck;
- tells you how you are doing;
- allows you to have your say;
- cares for your opinion;
- makes you feel clever;
- tells the truth.

Gardner (1993) considers the concept of multiple intelligences, one of which he defines as 'interpersonal intelligence' and which, in its advanced form, is 'the ability to read the intentions and desires – even when these have been hidden – of many individuals and, potentially, act upon this knowledge' (p. 240). I consider this would summarise the complexity of skills I had to develop as a teacher in order to advance the learning of my pupils.

What is the legislative framework that underpins your practice?

The legal framework within which teachers work is associated with rights and duties. Teachers have a variety of legal responsibilities, including:

- duty of care;
- health and safety;
- physical contact;
- detention of pupils;
- anti-discriminatory practice and human rights.

It is often the area of safeguarding children that requires the teacher to have a high degree of skills as a communicator in terms of listening and of responding through verbal and non-verbal means.

Case study

Pedro was a seven-year-old boy in my class who found reading difficult. He had an array of avoidance tactics that he would call on whenever reading was required of him. He had low self-esteem and genuinely believed he couldn't read or would ever be able to. His parents frequently came in to school to discuss his progress and were anxious that he should 'be able to read by now' and felt it was because he was lazy. I noticed that Pedro most enjoyed the times when he worked in a small informal group where he felt that he wasn't under pressure to perform. It was during these sessions that he often recalled the routine of how he was made to practise his reading at home, and that he was frequently sent to his room to bed without any tea if he couldn't remember all the words in his reading book. He said that nobody came to see him and he stayed there until the next morning. Sometimes his mum and dad got so angry they would smack him, and once his auntie was there and she told his dad to stop it.

The teacher's legal responsibilities in these situations are very clear. Under common law, the teacher has a 'duty of care' and is required to do all that is reasonable to protect the health, safety and welfare of pupils. The Children Act 1989 states that schools – and therefore teachers – have a duty to assist local authority social services departments to act on behalf of children in need or enquire into allegations of child abuse. The needs of the child are paramount. Under the Education Act 2002 schools have to take steps to protect children who are at risk from significant harm. Harm is defined as 'ill treatment, or impairment of a child's physical or mental health or of their physical, intellectual, emotional, social and behavioural development'.

It is during times like the ones mentioned above that children often disclose details of their home life and teachers have to consider the situation carefully. While I had to be a good listener and make sure I didn't ask leading questions, I was not qualified to make judgements. As a teacher, I had to be careful not to make promises of confidentiality when a child makes a disclosure, because teachers are legally obliged to share the information with the nominated person in the school who has responsibility for children's safeguarding, usually a senior member of staff. It is the nominated person's role to liaise with the relevant agencies, normally social services. While it was tempting to try to resolve this situation with the child and the parents myself, I had to remember the role of the teacher in this context and my legal responsibilities; this was regardless of the impact of my action on my relationship with parents.

What theoretical models underpin your practice?

I quickly realised that a child's ability to learn does not take place in a vacuum. Neither is their physical presence in the classroom and my interaction with them sufficient for optimum learning to take place. Maslow (1970) identified a hierarchy of individual needs that have to be met in order for humans to fulfil their true potential. This has been a useful frame of reference and has informed my practice considerably. Children cannot learn properly unless the following needs have been met, the first having to be met before the second and so forth:

- physical needs;
- being safe, both physically and emotionally;
- feeling of belonging;
- self-esteem;
- achieving true potential.

Case study

Robert often came to school hungry and tired. He had poor personal hygiene and had difficulty concentrating on class activities. He had special educational needs and was performing well below the standard expected of a 10-year-old. He had difficulty establishing relationships with the other children and frequently engaged in confrontation at lunch time. Some of the other children in the class were particularly hostile towards him, often being quick to accuse him of anything that had happened when someone had been hurt or things went missing. Sometimes

▶

Robert's tough shell would crumble and he would curl himself up in a corner of the classroom and sob uncontrollably. Attempts to discuss the situation with his parents had been relatively unsuccessful.

As a teacher, some of these factors were within my influence, while others were not. Knowing which of these I could influence with Robert was essential to working towards helping him to learn. Self-awareness and awareness of others are critical skills that I needed in this case. Goleman (1996) refers to these as some of the attributes of emotional intelligence. I had to be empathetic to Robert's needs, which Goleman defines as 'sensing others' feelings and perspective, and taking an active interest in their concerns'. People with this competence:

- are attentive to emotional cues and listen well;
- show sensitivity and understand others' perspectives;
- help out based on understanding other people's needs and feelings.

I arranged for Robert to attend the breakfast club at the school and assigned a teaching assistant to discreetly offer him a clean uniform as he arrived, should he need it. I sought to discover Robert's strengths, which turned out to be music and art, and ensured he was praised for these and given responsibility within the class to work with and help others in these subject areas. I also made sure he had extra support for aspects of the curriculum he found difficult and set tasks for him that he could see were achievable. I introduced the notion of the 'special day' where everyone had a turn and had certain privileges for the day. The highlight of this was a session which involved other classmates saying why they thought that person was special. This helped to raise Robert's self-esteem and helped more positive relationships to be established. I had to recognise that other professionals had to become involved with the parents as well as myself. Ultimately the family was allocated a social worker who monitored Robert's well-being and safety in the home.

What are the ethical issues that impact on your practice?

Teachers constantly face ethical challenges in the course of their practice and it is often difficult to separate them from moral ones. Arthur *et al.*

(2005) suggest that morality is about rules, principles and ideals, and ethics refers to the moral standards that apply to the teaching profession. They suggest that ethics for the teacher involves both attitude (which relates to the teacher's inner character or attitude as an ethical person) and action. The term ethics therefore refers to the characteristic values of a teacher. For a teacher, these ethical principles apply in a variety of contexts, including when working with pupils, parents/carers and professional colleagues.

Respect and fairness for all pupils have underpinned my practice throughout my teaching career and there have been times where I have had to challenge others when in my view these values have been compromised.

Case study

Mrs Brown, the lunchtime supervisor who looked after my class of six- and seven-year-olds, informed me she had kept the whole class in during lunch time because three pupils had misbehaved in the line and, as a consequence, it had taken a long time to escort them all to the dining hall. My interpretation was of the whole class of 30 being punished quite severely for the behaviour of three children. Some of the other children in the class complained bitterly that 'they had missed their playtime and they didn't do anything'. I understood Mrs Brown's frustration; her role was difficult and demanding. She had previously had difficulties with the three pupils in question. We discussed her feelings about the situation and she acknowledged she was exasperated and didn't know what else to do. It was important that I showed empathy and respect but, at the same time, encouraged self-reflection and awareness. When appropriate, I also challenged her respectfully.

Teachers work within a framework of legislation, statutory guidance and school policies and, while teachers do not have a code of ethics per se, they are bound by the Statement of Professional Values and Practice for Teachers that is underwritten by the General Teaching Council (GTC, 2006a) for England. Relevant to the above case study, the statement includes the following:

- Teachers treat young people fairly and with respect, take their views, opinions and feelings seriously and value diversity and individuality.
- Teachers see themselves as part of a team in securing the learning and well-being of young people.
- Teachers understand and respect the roles of other colleagues.

I felt I needed to address the notion of fairness, justice and respect from the pupils' perspective and from that of Mrs Brown. I was able to support Mrs Brown to use other strategies to manage pupil behaviour, including the use of rewards (stickers) for those who behaved appropriately in the line and the use of appropriate sanctions (which included missing playtime as well as others). I listened to the pupils' concerns and allowed them the opportunity to say how they felt. I then explored with them how they thought Mrs Brown must have felt. This was pursued further with the three boys in question privately away from the rest of the class. A consequence of this of course was for the rest of the class to express how they felt about the three boys. This led to further work using a solution-focused approach during circle time.

Working with people can be very demanding. How do you care for yourself?

The National Agreement on Raising Standards and Tackling Teacher Workload (ATL *et al.*, 2003) acknowledged that teachers and head teachers often have excessive workloads and gave recognition to the importance of a work-life balance. The National Union of Teachers (NUT, 1999, 2007) suggest that stress is one of the biggest problems facing teachers today and that teachers suffer more occupational stress then most other employees.

Case study

I remember arriving at school at 8 a.m. one day and taking a deep breath as I stepped onto the 'treadmill' as I went through the door, knowing it would be many hours before I would be able to 'get off'. I arrived early to finish my lesson planning and to locate the learning resources I was going to need. I had some pupils in the class who had challenging behaviour. They seemed to take up a lot of my time to the point where I often felt guilty that I was neglecting the others. At the end of the morning, over lunchtime, I had some records to write up and some children to see individually to give them some extra time hearing them read. I

---

ate my lunch 'on the hoof'. When lunchtime was over I still hadn't finished writing up all the records. In the afternoon, there was a great deal of excitement and noise in the class because it was a special art afternoon which the children loved, but it took a lot of organising, particularly as there were four different activities going on in the classroom at once. Even though the children helped with the clearing up, it was hectic and I had to oversee it carefully to ensure everything was done in a safe and orderly manner. At the end of the day, there were reading books and homework to sort out for the children to take home. Once the children had gone, I took the opportunity to finish writing up my records and started to write my evaluations of the day's lessons. At 4.30 p.m. I rushed off to another school to attend a twilight course that finished at 6 p.m. I finally stepped down from my 'treadmill' and went home. In the evening I finished writing up my lesson evaluations and reflected on whether I was adequately meeting the learning needs of all the children in my class. This stayed on my mind all evening.

Clearly there are many stress factors in this example, not all of which can be avoided, but it is how they are managed that influences our ability to cope with stress. Maintaining a healthy work–life balance is a challenge when working in a profession that involves people. As a teacher I felt torn and very often agreed to things because they were of benefit to the pupils, but didn't consider whether it would be good for me. The Teacher Support Network (TSN, 2007) suggests teachers try to adopt coping strategies, some of which include:

- taking personal responsibility for work–life balance, which includes speaking up when work expectations and demands are too much;
- working smart, not long, which involves prioritising and trying not to get caught up in non-productive activities;
- taking proper breaks;
- ensuring there is a line drawn between work and leisure;
- recognising the importance of exercise, leisure and friendships.

Eventually, I did adopt some of these strategies. I made better use of computer systems to keep my records up to date and delegated some of this responsibility under my direction to the teaching assistant. I made sure I had spent at least 20 minutes at lunchtime sitting down in the staffroom eating lunch and chatting with colleagues. I avoided as much as possible taking work home on weekday evenings although I still had some to do at weekends. I also joined a gym and made sure I went twice a week after school.

How do you ensure your practice responds to current research?

As a teacher, while developing a community of learning within the classroom, I also needed to be part of a learning community myself. It was important to keep up to date with current research on curriculum developments and the way children learn. All qualified teachers who are teaching in maintained and non-maintained schools are required to register with the GTC, the teachers' regulatory body. The GTC strongly encourages teachers to keep up to date with research. From my own experience, this was always most beneficial when it was discussed and reflected on with other colleagues.

I was teaching young children at the time and became very interested in the new research that confirmed the value of young children's learning being enhanced by being outdoors. I had become aware of the research related to this in a number of ways, including reading books and journal articles, reading publications from the Department for Education and Skills (DfES) [now the Department for Children, Schools and Families (DCSF)] and watching the relevant programmes on Teachers TV. I decided I wanted to investigate further. I shared views and exchanged research evidence and related publications at our local cluster group meeting with other schools in the area. This led to us setting up our own mini-research project into the impact of outdoor provision on children's learning. We also shared ideas on how best to set up outdoor provision, the resources that would be required and how the curriculum would be delivered outside. This became a **longitudinal** study based within action research and was constantly informed by other related research in the public domain. It required convincing the senior members of staff of the value of the research and being allowed to be creative and take risks. Ultimately the research had a genuine impact on practice.

The GTC (2006b) considers that the research engagement of teachers needs to adhere to the following core principles if it is to have an impact on practice.

- It has to be focused on school improvement.
- It is about improving teaching and learning.
- It is shared among all staff.
- It is supported by school leaders and governors.
- It is seen as a professional development activity.

- It is used for educational decision making.
- It is embedded in school systems and culture.
- It is a platform for the development of learning communities, both within and outside the school.
- It is an opportunity for collective reflection on **pedagogy**, assessment, curriculum and leadership.
- It can be involvement in large and small research projects.
- It is a link between schools and education policy.

With the advent of the world wide web, teachers have access to research they never had before and the DCSF Standards website now has a research-informed practice portal whose aim is 'to help make sure that practice and policy in schools, and at a regional and national level, are informed by good and up-to-date evidence'. This site takes articles from research journals and summarises them and groups the research according to themes. These include new digests of the latest research from research journals, new information about current research being undertaken, news and views from special interest groups, ongoing discussion and feedback and links to a range of related sites and resources, and can be found at **www.standards.dfes.gov.uk/research.**

How are your continuing professional development needs fulfilled?

Continuing professional development (CPD) was important to me at all stages in my teaching career, although I had different needs at different points. The Training and Development Agency (TDA, 2007a) for schools defines CPD as consisting of 'a reflective activity designed to improve an individual's attributes, knowledge, understanding and skills. It supports individual needs and improves professional practice' (p. 2).

In the past it was called in-service training (INSET) and had an emphasis on what was being delivered rather than the outcome. However, Gray (2005) suggests that the change in terminology shifted the emphasis away from the provider towards the individual. Gray also points out that the term CPD does not differentiate between learning from courses and learning on the job.

When I was asked to take over the responsibility for special educational needs in the school where I was teaching I realised that, while all teachers are teachers of children with special educational needs, I needed to ensure I was secure enough in my knowledge and skills to support other staff within the school and update my own expertise. With the support of the head teacher of my school, I enrolled on a course being run by the local education authority over a period of a few months. This proved to be really useful, as it acknowledged the knowledge and skills I already had and built on them further. It was an opportunity to reflect with other colleagues from different schools and it became a problem-solving forum. The ongoing nature of the course enabled me to go back into school, implement some of the things I had learned and share them with the rest of the staff. After the course had finished I found I had become more confident in my own ability and it had fuelled a thirst for further development of my knowledge and skills. Subsequently I enrolled on a Masters in Education in Special Needs at a university nearby. This enabled me to have an even greater degree of control over my own learning which subsequently influenced the rest of my career in education.

In recent years there has been greater investment in teachers' professional learning through a variety of initiatives. According to the GTC (2007), the more influence teachers have over their professional development, the more likely they are to find it effective. The TDA (2007b) cite the following as examples of CPD activities that a teacher may engage in:

- professional development meetings and professional development items in staff and team meetings;
- attending external conferences and courses;
- attending internal conferences and courses and professional development events;
- coaching and mentoring, shadowing and peer support;
- participating in networks or projects;
- lesson observations;
- discussions with colleagues or pupils to reflect on working practices;
- research and investigation.

As a busy teacher, there were often ideas I had thought about but hadn't got round to putting into practice. CPD helped provide the space for reflection and to make some of the ideas happen. In my own experience head teachers and senior staff played a crucial role in making CPD happen and in making it effective. They were the ones who led a school culture that valued openly the professional learning of everyone by encouraging the sharing of professional knowledge.

How do you manage the conflicting demands of working with service users, colleagues and managers?

Most teachers would recognise that it is they as a person who has the most impact on their ability to teach. Prosser (1999) suggests there are emotional costs of sustaining the interpersonal relationships that give teachers some of their main job satisfactions and that this also provides many of their main pressures and anxieties. As a teacher it was important to develop safety mechanisms and self-help strategies to help me cope with the conflicting demands placed on me.

Case study

One busy week during the autumn term I had a number of demands on me, all of which required my attention within the week.

- Three pupils were exhibiting a lot of attention-seeking behaviour which was getting in the way of their own learning and the learning of others.
- I had received some reports of bullying from some children in my class and a complaint had been made by one of the parents who had asked to see me to discuss the matter.
- I was conscious that a newly qualified teacher who I had been mentoring had been having a few difficulties recently and was in need of my support.
- I had been asked by the head teacher to talk to the governors about the proposed new special educational needs policy.

I usually came into school early in the morning and found this was the best time for me to engage in high-quality thinking with few disturbances or distractions. It was also a time to talk things through with colleagues and share ideas. I talked through the attention-seeking behaviour with colleagues and together we came up with some strategies I could try. I made a note of these so I could refer to them later if I needed to. My reflection time also enabled me to carefully consider my approach to the bullying issue, with both the parents and the children concerned. It was important to make sure I knew I would be supported on whatever approach I decided to take, so I consulted with the head teacher.

I knew that I had to prioritise the demands on me and set myself a plan. I set up a meeting with the newly qualified teacher after school, ensuring it was on a day I had no other commitments after school. I also set up a firm start time and a finish time; this helped to keep the discussion focused. The meeting with the governors had been in my diary for some time so I had planned ahead and was already well on the way to being prepared for the meeting by the time the week came.

Bartell (2005) considers that teaching was once regarded as an isolated profession where teachers worked autonomously in the classroom. More recently this is changing and there is much more of a culture of collaboration. In research carried out by Prosser (1999) teachers' interpersonal relationships with colleagues took precedence over their bureaucratic activities at all levels. As a result teachers felt responsible for one another as people and were mutually answerable for the work of the whole school. I think my own experience would support this view. I gained much emotional and professional support from colleagues, even as an experienced teacher.

Bubb and Earley (2004) advocate the importance of teachers planning ahead and prioritising. I have to admit that my first priority was always to the pupils in my class, partially because I felt this was a moral and professional responsibility, but also because this was usually where most emotional energy was expended and perhaps, as Nias (1989) points out, the teachers' relationship with the pupil is so central to the way they see themselves as people and practitioners.

Conclusion

Teachers often find it hard to separate themselves from their role as a teacher and themselves as just human beings. Consequently, the emotional demands as well as professional demands are great. In order for a teacher to be effective and maintain a healthy well-being, the development of good interpersonal skills is crucial. Teachers' interactions are multilayered and often complex, communicating with different audiences with different needs, sometimes at the same time, sometimes at different times. A question that is often asked is whether teachers are born or made? I would argue both. There is no doubt that some teachers already possess a high degree of interpersonal skills that seem to be inbuilt, but all teachers can learn and develop these skills further. In my own experience it seems this is best done through shared reflection in a number of environments, including through continuing professional development, through discussion with colleagues and sometimes, where appropriate, in reflection with pupils. Teachers who are effective communicators do this within a secure backdrop of knowledge related to their legal and ethical obligations as well as their knowledge of how children learn and factors that influence this. Teachers also do this by keeping up to date with current issues and research and sharing knowledge with each other.

Key learning points

- Teachers' interactions are multilayered and often complex: communicating with different audiences with different needs, sometimes at the same time, sometimes at different times.
- Teachers who are effective communicators do so within a secure backdrop of knowledge related to their legal and ethical obligations, as well as their knowledge of how children learn and factors that influence this.
- The emotional demands as well as the professional demands are great. In order for a teacher to be effective and maintain a healthy well-being, the development of good interpersonal skills is crucial.
- Shared reflection in a number of environments including through discussion with colleagues and sometimes, where appropriate, in reflection with pupils is essential for the CPD of a teacher.

REFLECTION ACTIVITIES

1. How would you define a 'good' teacher, taking into account what you have just read?
2. Are some interpersonal skills more important for a teacher than others?
3. Do you think the interpersonal skills teachers need to develop will be different according to the type of school in which they teach?
4. A question that is often asked is whether teachers are born or made. Think about your own experiences of teachers. Which do you think is most likely?

FURTHER READING

Arthur, J., Davison, J. and Lewis, M.(2005) *Professional Values and Practice: Achieving the Standards for QTS*. London: RoutledgeFalmer

DfES (2005) *Primary National Strategy: Relationships in the Classroom*. See: **www.standards.dfes.gov.uk/primary/publications/banda/1086075/** (accessed 14 February 2008)

Goleman, D. (1996) *Emotional Intelligence. Why It Can Matter More Than IQ*. London: Bloomsbury

Chapter 3

Interpersonal Skills in the Police Service

David Collicott

EDITOR'S INTRODUCTION

In this chapter David discusses how members of the police service, both officers and **police staff,** use interpersonal skills. You will see how the demands and needs of both the public and staff members can be similar but also vastly different. In our increasingly multicultural society police officers are expected to deal with anything and everything in a sensitive and appropriate manner.

In one day an officer might, among other things, have to tell someone that their loved one has died, spend time with someone accused of murder, quell a violent, alcohol-fuelled fight and deal with a perpetrator and victim of domestic abuse. In addition each day an officer may be putting his or her own life at risk to protect the community that they serve. The case studies demonstrate the challenges of such a varied remit.

Key themes

- Diversity.
- Dealing with those whose behaviour is unacceptable.
- Values.
- Non-judgemental approach.
- Individual need.
- Behavioural adjustment.

DAVID COLLICOTT – POLICE OFFICER

The 'modern' police service, as created by Sir Robert Peel in 1829, never stops developing and the introduction of new legislation and changing responsibilities mean that those employed within the service have to develop and update their skills regularly. Underlying all of this is the fact that police service staff interact with people both inside and outside the service on a daily basis. It will become evident that one communication tool is not sufficient in all circumstances. A range of skills is required and they need to be used flexibly, according to the demands and needs of the client. For the purposes of this discussion the term 'client' is used to describe anyone that I come into contact with within my work role and this includes perpetrators, victims and colleagues.

As there is no direct entry into senior ranks of the police service, all officers must train and work as constables before seeking promotion. This gives every police officer the opportunity to learn 'on the job' by dealing with the wide-ranging demands of the community. In common with all other officers I have worked in both operational and support roles, which have added to my skills base.

Describe the kind of interactions that you might have with people in the course of a normal working day

My current post is in Traffic Management and Road Safety. I oversee all fatal road collisions and manage many of the staff who deal with both the incident and the families involved. The variety of skills that are used within the police service is wide-ranging. A non-exhaustive list would include:

- adviser;
- fixer;
- supporter;
- negotiator;
- helper;

- assessor;
- counsellor;
- trainer;
- mentor;
- enforcer;
- controller;
- discipliner;
- defuser;
- debriefer.

Some of these skills will be obvious, but others may be less familiar or not customarily linked with members of police service staff. These will be explained through this chapter.

In general terms interactions take place in three areas: internal, external agencies/partners and the public. While similar skills can be used with all these groups a clear awareness is necessary of how each group's needs differs as this affects how best to deal with them. The types of interactions follow the three ego states described by Berne (1961) – Parent, Adult and Child – within the transactional analysis (TA) model. Transactions and responses can take place among any of the levels but it will depend on the participants and the particular circumstances whether the interaction can be categorised as complementary, crossed or ulterior/covert.

A complementary transaction between two people would be where the response comes 'from the ego state the transaction was aimed at' (see Figure 1) but where this goes wrong 'it is called a crossed transaction' (Donnelly and Neville, 2008, pp. 42–3). There are nine types of complementary interactions, but 'Berne (1972) calculated there were mathematically 72 types of crossed interactions' (Donnelly and Neville, 2008, p. 44). This indicates that there are eight times as many opportunities for a transaction to receive a response from a different ego state than that intended.

In internal interactions the skills can include the complete range listed above, depending on the post or role that the individual is undertaking and the specifics of the interaction. Working with external agencies or partners is less likely to involve any of the enforcement or control activities but will involve negotiator, helper and fixer skills more frequently.

When assisting members of the public who have been victims of crime or subjects of other incidents such as Road Traffic Collisions (RTC), the skills will be supportive, helping to resolve problems or provide information. Clearly, this differs from dealing with those who are alleged offenders, which will involve skills including enforcement and controlling.

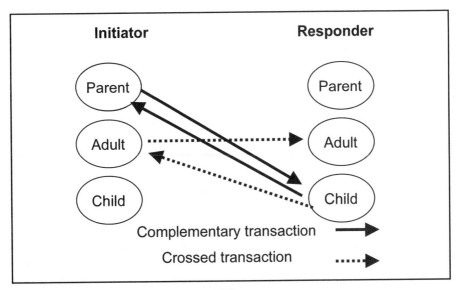

Figure 1 Crossed transactions (Berne, 1972)

There is often an expectation from the public that 'The Police' will fix anything and everything. For a young constable this can be a difficult expectation to match. Natural resilience, knowledge and flexibility are key attributes to develop, alongside practical skills. Interpersonal skills cannot only be developed and honed through training and practical use.

Often the police service is called upon to resolve issues that are the responsibility of other agencies but, due to the time of day (or night), these agencies are not available. Knowledge of how to console the caller, provide them with access to the necessary support and assist with the immediate needs is essential.

Case study

An elderly lady whose water pipe burst during a Saturday evening called the police as the local council offices were shut. I attended, resolved her immediate need by turning off the water but could not fix the burst pipe. Through the Control Room I obtained the details and made contact with the Council's emergency service. Having explained that the water was no longer flooding the house the Council were considering calling on the following Monday. Through clarifying the lady's situation and using some persuasion the operator agreed to arrange for the repair to be made later that day.

▶

> Without the immediate fix there would have been even worse flooding and the lady's home and life would have been adversely affected. It is always satisfying to resolve a crisis and leave a job knowing that somebody's life has been improved through your work. Trainers, tutors and mentors have an important part to play in the development of these types of ability in their trainees.

Considering the significant age gap in this case I had taken the role of the Parent and the lady that of the Child, as I was guiding and advising her. As she did not have any means to resolve her problems herself her responses were also as a Child to my Parent status. My interactions with the Council had started as Adult to Adult, but moved to Parent to Adult when I had to explain the specific needs of the situation, and then back to Adult/Adult. While this migration between the ego states was not obvious during the interaction it became clear when reviewing the conversations. During this incident the transactions were all complementary, even when they migrated between the different ego statuses.

As a police supervisor and manager I use a range of skills to resolve issues, and help, develop and support my staff and colleagues on an individual or an organisational basis. As a Critical Incident Stress Debriefer I have carried out debriefs of staff involved in local incidents including fatal RTC and firearms incidents and those who have returned from deployments with the International Policing Units in Bosnia, Afghanistan and East Timor.

It is often asked by outsiders why we provide a high level of emotional support to our staff because they often believe that all police officers have personal strengths above those of the 'ordinary' person. While most officers are normally able to separate themselves from the stresses and emotional pressures there are times when personal circumstances reduce their capacity to deal with a particular problem. Employers, not just the police service, have a legal duty of care for their staff. This was first emphasised in the court case of *Walker* v. *Northumberland County Council* (1995) which raised the need for psychological as well as physical care. While 'Everly and Mitchell have emphasized that by debriefing individuals following severe traumatic events, organizations can reduce risk of law-suits' (McNally *et al.*, 2003. p. 74), there is an ethical aspect that providing such care is more of a necessity.

What are the key skills that you use in your work with people?

The types of skills I use will depend on the type of person with whom I am interacting. The skills can often change during the interaction and will frequently overlap. It is never simply treating all offenders in one way and victims in another. Both may require a level of counselling and also control. The underlying principle I use is that depicted in Betari's box (see Figure 2).

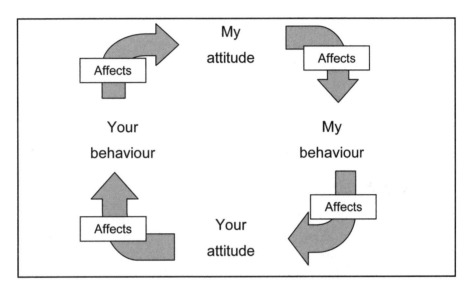

Figure 2 Betari's box (Clements and Jones, 2006, p. 182)

The phrase to 'fail the attitude test' is often used in relation to the reaction of those accused of committing an offence who, when confronted, become agitated, argumentative or aggressive. Occasionally, this can be due to the attitude and behaviour of the officer, displaying some form of prejudice towards the individual or, more often, a reaction to the offender's attitude and behaviour. When the Betari model is applied this shows that the attitude and behaviour can result in a negative change which, if not stopped, will continue to worsen. During training police officers and police staff who are in direct contact with the public receive inputs relating to action/reaction. The basis is to ensure that the initial contact is made in a calm and non-inflammatory manner so that no adverse behavioural traits are displayed and any reaction is at a reasonable level. However, when other factors such as alcohol are involved, any such attempt can be pointless but ensures that the officer maintains emotional, attitudinal and behavioural control. While working within custody I have had arrested persons presented who have displayed aggressive behaviour as normally shown by drunken people. When further checks have been made I have found that they have been suffering from a medical condition or injury. I can never assume that a displayed behaviour is the same as the person's attitude.

The operational constable, for a significant part of their working hours, will be with members of the public who have been victims. Having provided support and assistance to a victim they could then be called on to deal with offenders. This might be in the initial stages, making an arrest before handing over to specialists from the Criminal Investigation Department (CID) or other units, or dealing with the offender through the whole investigation process. This means that there is a need to be able to change styles easily and appropriately.

Dealing with the public requires most interactions to be formal and correct; a victim does not expect an officer to be emotionally involved in their problem. They count on the officer to provide support to them at their time of need. Likewise, when dealing with an offender, there is a need for them to be dealt with so that evidence is gathered correctly without emotions or personal preferences to affect them. That does not mean, however, that the officer should be stand-offish, abrupt or rude. It is a delicate balance, differing from case to case and according to the individual, and can change on a daily basis. There are several offenders whom I have dealt with on the streets and in the cells whom I have also met at other non-work-related times. I have maintained a sociable approach that has been reflected by these former clients. Police officers are subject to strict discipline and 'consorting with criminals' is not acceptable. That does not mean that you cannot be friendly and approachable.

So how is an officer expected to deal with a victim?

Case study

While I was a local beat officer, attending both emergency calls and follow-up enquiries, I was called to the home of a middle-aged couple who returned from an evening out and found that their house had been burgled. This was not a particularly unusual event but the level of disturbance was. The burglar had ransacked almost all of the rooms, turning out drawers and strewing the contents around the rooms. Large items had been smashed and smaller things stolen. The contents of the fridge had been thrown across the kitchen and, due to the time delay, had congealed into a multicoloured mess. This was a very unpleasant end to an evening out that was made worse due to it being in the lead up to Christmas and almost all the presents had been taken from under the tree.

This type of event requires the police officer to provide support and empathy ('recognising and acknowledging someone's feelings without necessarily feeling them yourself' (Thompson, 2006, p. 132)) for the victims while ensuring that the best evidence is gathered. This can be difficult as victims need to come to terms with what has happened to them while being subjected to some restrictions.

I spent time explaining the various processes of how evidence would be gathered and the need to preserve various areas for forensic examination, so controlling the victims in one room for as much time as possible. For the victim this can be very hard, as they will want to get their home back to 'normal'. Clear reasons for the request have to be explained and this can take some time. This often raises issues with the control room who have other incidents requiring attendance. Officers have to justify their continuing engagement at some incidents causing personal conflicts.

My interactions with the couple were on an Adult to Adult basis, providing information and guidance at a level that was suitable for them. Although they were understandably traumatised they did not move to the Child ego status, which would have required me to amend my approach to accommodate this, even when providing additional information.

Awareness of personal, religious or other restrictions helps to ensure that police work is carried out with sensitivity. In a burglary case involving a Muslim family I needed to use a police dog to track where the offender had gone. Knowing that it is offensive to Muslims to have a dog in their home I explained our needs and was able to take the dog into the rear yard through a neighbour's property. This had a detrimental effect on the dog's effectiveness due to the time delay but ensured that the family were not subjected to further distress.

Personal needs also have to be considered when a person is in custody having been arrested for allegedly committing an offence. When dealing with an alleged offender the investigating officer will prepare a plan based on the PEACE Interview Model (Keogh, 2007), which advocates the development of a 'proper relationship between the interviewer and interviewee. This requires, for example, that the officer develops an awareness of, and is able to respond to, the welfare needs of the interviewee and any particular fears and expectations.' Some of this awareness will be obtained through the alleged offender's legal adviser or the custody staff, but it still requires the officer to interact with the person directly. The interaction is cessary to ensure that some form of response is received during the interview. The same type of knowledge of people's needs, 'physiological' and 'safety' as described by Abraham Maslow, is essential to ensure that these do not impinge on the ability to carry out interviews. Legal restrictions, as included in the Police and Criminal Evidence Act, relate to the care of persons in custody and how they are treated and dealt with during interview. However, even where the interaction is at its best, the interview may result in the alleged offender giving no comment to the questions posed.

Case study

During my earlier career I was working with the custody officer. A man in his late 60s was arrested for killing his daughter. The daughter had been severely disabled from birth and was unable to do anything unaided. Together with his wife the man had provided care for her for over 40 years. This had placed an immense strain on the couple, who had worked as a team to provide 24-hour care for their daughter with little external assistance. The man's wife had died about a month prior to his arrest and he had found the daily demands on him to be excessive. He had either not sought or been unable to access any of the support services that could help and he had become so desperate that he had smothered his daughter while she slept.

In the general public's viewpoint murderers are seen as being callous and heartless people and should be dealt with firmly and without compassion. In this case the man had reached the extreme of his capacity to deal both with grief and the daily demands of caring for his daughter. He had seen no other way to cope with the demands. He had been completely open about what he had done, unlike the general perception of murderers. Before his first interview I was detailed to sit with him as there were concerns that he might harm himself. A social worker was called and took on the responsibility of 'appropriate adult' for the interview process.

Throughout, the man had sat quietly, only seeking an occasional drink of water. Our interactions were always on the Parent/Child ego status basis as he had no knowledge of police procedures and he had a need for some emotional support which, along with practical support since his wife's death, had been unmet. He was a 'normal' person driven to take a desperate action and was treated without prejudice or contempt.

Case study

Police Community Support Officer (PCSO) Aziz had finished training for his new post only six months ago and had been on solo patrol for three weeks before being detailed to attend a complaint of a group of youths causing a nuisance outside a small shopping centre. He recognised a few of the youths and went to speak with them, hoping to resolve the incident through persuasion on an Adult/Adult basis. All started well. When others arrived the group started to joke around the officer. One of the new youths then grabbed PCSO Aziz's uniform cap from his head. PCSO Aziz attempted to grab it back but the youth ran off, dropping the cap on a nearby waste bin. This shows a change of the interaction to that of the Child/Child status and, while this could be seen by many as a trivial piece of tomfoolery, PCSO Aziz was shocked by the behaviour.

Once I was aware of what had happened I knew that there was a need to support and reassure PCSO Aziz. I met with him. Following the steps of defusing I started out by asking him to explain what had happened and how he felt, maintaining the Adult/Adult status. He told me that something similar had recently taken place with another PCSO and that he felt that the incident was not racially motivated. (If the incident had been considered as racially motivated it would have required a full investigation.)

I asked about his expectations and ambitions. He stated his intention to carry on being a PCSO and to make a difference in his community. He explained that during his first weeks on patrol he had been welcomed, made to feel an integral part of the unit and the community and that he wanted to continue to build on that start.

▶

It was clear he had lost his confidence and that the main need was to provide support to help him return to his full duties. The main criterion was to ensure that he did not feel demeaned or consider himself to have failed. Adopting a Parent/Adult approach I encouraged him to consider what options were possible and which he felt most comfortable with.

I also considered how the two incidents were likely to provoke 'defence mechanisms' as identified by Sigmund Freud (1894). His theory is that these mechanisms are developed and learned in response to triggers, the steps to these triggers being the 'perception' of a problem, 'analysis' and 'decision-making'.

We agreed that to achieve the objective he would benefit from the support of a mentor. I contacted an experienced PCSO and provided them with a briefing on the expectations of the mentoring. I asked PCSO Aziz to make a diary of events and incidents that he attended with the mentor and to discuss how they had dealt with them, including how he felt. Initially, the mentoring was planned to run for a month with us meeting each week. However, with the additional support he was given and through the use of his diary, after only three weeks PCSO Aziz had returned to solo patrol and was interacting with youngsters with confidence again. I have spoken with him on several occasions since and he says that he continues to use the diary. He includes in it things that have gone well to reassure himself and those that have gone less well with some considerations for different approaches for the future.

As a manager I have to be aware of the organisation's legal and ethical responsibilities to the well-being of its staff. Anybody who is involved with a traumatic incident is likely to require some form of support. The range of the support will differ according to the specific aspects of the incident, how the staff member was involved and the individual's specific needs.

Case study

Control Room Operator Jenny was on duty when a road traffic collision occurred, which resulted in the death of the man driver and serious injuries to his young child. This was before the network of family liaison officers (FLO) was established. Through enquiries carried out by local officers it was discovered that the dead man's wife was working in another part of the country. It was necessary to make contact with the wife and bring her back to the hospital where the child was in the intensive therapy unit (ITU). I gave Jenny the task of making contact with the local police to arrange for an officer to attend the wife's workplace. She had to review all of the information on the incident log and prepare how she could relay this first to the other force in order to make the arrangements and then to the officers who were going to attend. She also contacted the company to seek their assistance in providing a suitable room and support for the woman. Throughout these contacts additional information was being added to the incident log including details of injuries and background to the crash. This meant that Jenny was exposed to and had to pass on this information several times without becoming emotionally involved.

I kept direct contact with Jenny, ensuring that she was comfortable with everything she was being asked to do and that she had all of the information she needed. At the end of the incident I carried out a defusing session with Jenny. 'Defusing is about showing officers that emotions like anger, bitterness, denial and guilt are normal feelings to have following a traumatic incident' (Mulraney, 2001) and is normally provided on a one-to-one or as 'a small group intervention – within 12 hours' (McNally *et al.*, 2003, p. 53). This is more in-depth than a general discussion and is intended to ensure that in the event of some emotional upset they are 'experiencing a perfectly normal reaction to a terrible event' (Mulraney, 2001, p. 32).

I established how she had felt at the time and how she felt now. The end of the session was to ensure that she was fully aware of the additional support she could call on, whether through me or the other sources in both the Control Room department and from the rest of the Constabulary.

The level of support provided to staff members is dependent on the specific type of incident. Any incident involving fatalities will automatically raise the potential of a full critical incident stress debrief (CISD).

Case study

Sergeant Woods was the first officer at the scene of another road traffic collision. In the car was a boy aged nine years who was unresponsive, his mother who was seriously injured and the boy's two elder sisters who were uninjured. Sergeant Woods attempted, along with an off-duty nurse, to resuscitate the boy. They continued, assisting the paramedics until the boy was removed to hospital. The boy was declared dead some time after arrival at hospital after the medical team had continued the attempts to revive him.

Sergeant Woods had a son of a similar age and was adversely affected by the incident and was unfit to work for several days. It was the responsibility of the managers to look after their staff welfare issues, generally without any specific training to ensure that this was carried out effectively.

While he was away from work I kept regular contact with him to ensure that he had no immediate needs for other support. As there were none I arranged to meet with him on his return to work. At this meeting we went through a form of defusing session similar to the one I used with Jenny. However, in this instance it was obvious that Sergeant Woods had been emotionally affected by the collision and his involvement. Knowing that his needs were beyond my capabilities I made arrangements for him to speak with the Welfare Officer and then with the independent counselling service. Some time later we were both invited to a formal debriefing session that was arranged by the NHS as there had been a number of staff within the A&E department, as well as the paramedics, who had been involved with trying to save the boy's life. This was conducted by a trained debriefer.

At this time this was a new concept that has been introduced to deal with those who have been involved in a critical incident.

In my current role as a senior investigating officer (SIO) for road deaths I am the lead for investigations, guiding the officer in charge (OIC) and others, for example collision investigators and the FLO, as to which areas to take into consideration. I also act as a review officer for other SIOs' investigations. This helps to ensure that all potential avenues of enquiry are followed. In doing so I occasionally identify areas that have not been considered or not included in the policy log. I then provide feedback to the SIO. This is normally as a face-to-face meeting but occasionally through a written memo. The information has to be delivered carefully, concisely and constructively. As these are peer reviews rather than assessments or appraisals the 'feedback sandwich' (where contentious issues to be discussed are sandwiched between more positive feedback points) is not generally used.

As a manager I have to deal with staff with sensitivity ensuring that any adverse comments are supported by evidence not supposition. At the same time I have a responsibility to the organisation to ensure that all the employees are working to their best capacity, so any poor performance issues have to be brought to the staff member's attention as soon as possible. Where there is a potential for disciplinary action any formal meetings are generally with the staff member's union or staff association representative.

The performance development review (PDR) is the organisation's mechanism for assessing a staff member's performance. Previously these were carried out purely as end-of-year appraisals. In recent years this has developed to a whole-year process by which evidence is gathered and recorded with quarterly reviews and monthly informal evaluations.

Case study

PC Williams had completed her probationary period and was working on follow-up enquiries on my area. There was a clear process for completing enquiries in a timely manner in order to achieve legal and quality requirements. During one month several of her enquiries were returned for amendment but, in her PDR evidence when I carried out a quarterly review, I found that she claimed that she had completed work to the required standard. I raised it at our meeting, referring to the evidence I had from the work control sheets and information given to me by other supervisors. The discussion was intense and difficult to manage, as she believed that her work was good. By having the evidence

▶

> available and clear I was able to demonstrate how her claims were unfounded. I then worked to find a way to encourage her to improve her workload and quality. Through action planning with regular reviews, following the SMARTER (Specific objectives that are Measurable, Achievable, Relevant, Time-limited, Evaluated and Reviewed) principles, and with the assistance of a mentor, PC Williams' work improved and her later PDR entries were accurately based.

While this example demonstrates that some assessment is based on slightly historic information I prefer to assess and provide feedback on a more contemporaneous basis and consider it to be 'the backbone of good **supervision**' (Dohrenwend, 2002, p. 43). By providing feedback I am able to reinforce the behaviour I 'want the employee to keep' and highlight and help identify behaviour I 'want the employee to change' (Dohrenwend, 2002, p. 43).

Using the 'feedback sandwich', where the assessor places the discussion of the negative trait between examples of good work, often helps to make a meeting easier to manage. However, when mismanaged or overused it can lead to a loss of confidence by the staff member. 'The main ingredient of a feedback sandwich is constructive criticism. When it is well timed, well targeted and well said, constructive criticism can help direct growth, motivate staff and offer relief from confusion' (Dohrenwend, 2002, p. 44).

What is the legislative framework which underpins your practice?

The police service is subject to a variety of legislation that imposes restrictions affecting particularly how officers interact with members of the public. There is a regular source of complaints based on the Police Code of Professional Standards. Among the most common complaints are those relating to incivility. This clearly relates to how police officers interact with the public and will often be during the points of contact when there are conflicts involved. However, there are occasions when this relates to dealing with victims. Again, there is guidance for what should be provided to victims and this is covered within the Victim's Charter 1996.

Police officers are not employees and therefore the Health and Safety at Work Act 1974 was not fully applicable to them. However, many of the requirements regarding the care and conditions of this Act were introduced by the Police (Health and Safety) Act 1997.

The Police and Criminal Evidence Act 1984 (PACE) and related Codes of Practice govern how offenders are dealt with and cared for during detention and investigations.

In a similar way the Road Deaths Investigation Manual 2007 (RDIM) and the Murder Investigation Manual 2006 (MIM) provide clear guidance relating to the procedures and expectations placed on investigators during major investigations. The principles are also transferable to other types of investigations.

What are the theoretical models that underpin your practice?

A range of theoretical models inform and underpin my practice. These are discussed in depth throughout the text and include:

- Betari's box;
- SMARTER principles;
- transactional analysis;
- Maslow's hierarchy of needs;
- PEACE interview model.

What are the ethical issues that impact on your practice?

A key factor that underlies any incident that we attend in the police service is the need for confidentiality. While 'confidentiality generally implies an element of trust to keep secret that which is disclosed to a person or persons and usually pertains to private and personal information' (Cuthbert and Quallington, 2008, p. 89) when dealing with my staff I make it clear that some information may have to be brought to the attention of others. Police officers are subject to a tightly restrictive series of regulations and a disclosed breach of these has to be investigated. Similarly, where I am unable to provide for all the apparent needs of the individual, I would have to seek assistance from another. In order to do this I would normally seek their agreement to me passing the details to the other person.

Where any interaction reveals any form of criminal offence I am required to deal with it in the same way as if I detected an offender on the street and according to the requirements of PACE.

For post-incident stress debriefs anything that is pertinent to the investigation would have to be disclosed to the investigating officer. Likewise, had the man who murdered his daughter spoken about certain points of what had happened, I would have written these onto his custody record as they could have been important to the investigation and could have been significant statements, disclosable to the court.

Working with people can be very demanding. How do you care for yourself?

The main need that I have is not allowing what I have seen or been involved with to affect my personal life. This can be difficult when those involved have similarities to your own circle of family and friends or when an incident occurs on a personally relevant day. I once attended a sudden death report on my birthday. Fortunately the circumstances, while unpleasant and in some ways tragic, were completely dissimilar to my own. In contrast, the death of a young boy who had suffered from a heart problem was more poignant, as he was of a similar age to my son. When I returned home the first thing I did was to give him a hug.

My main coping strategy is to speak about any incidents with either my colleagues or my wife. I am careful about the type of detail I share, either due to the confidentiality or the level of injuries that have been involved. However, I have found it key to my well-being to ensure that my life returns to 'normal' as quickly as possible. I also find that doing normal things, such as DIY, gardening, going for a long walk, cycling or swimming, help.

I have accepted the offer of attending debrief sessions following critical incidents. Also, as an SIO and FLO, I receive annual mental health checks with the Force Occupational Health Unit where any issues can be discussed.

How do you ensure that your practice responds to current research?

New or updated information regarding practices and procedures are published through the force weekly bulletins. These provide a certain level of detail. However, where legislation is concerned we have access to the National Legal database. While this covers criminal law primarily, it does provide a certain level of information regarding other legislation.

News and magazine articles that are highlighted through general browsing or through the various networking services also provide information. To supplement or extend the information I use the internet and professional journals, e.g. *Police Review*, *Police* and *Police Professional*, which have articles and source information.

In relation to the investigation and support for victims of RTCs I benefit from attending conferences and training seminars where case studies and new approaches are discussed. Her Majesty's Inspectorate of Constabulary (HMIC) undertakes thematic inspections of police forces. From these inspections examples of best practice are identified and included within the published reports.

How are your continuing professional development needs fulfilled?

For the majority of police service staff there are specific training programmes that support development either in specialisation or advancement. In recent years there has been a vast expansion of programmes that have been made available through the use of information systems (IS). The extension of access through the internet to the National Centre for Applied Learning Technologies (NCALT) programmes means that a variety of learning programmes can be completed without the need to attend a training venue.

I have access to various national conferences and seminars relating to Road Death Investigations and care for the bereaved relatives. These are organised by the National Policing Improvement Agency (NPIA), Brake and RoadPeace and involve practitioners from a range of professions.

For FLO we run in-force courses to keep up to date with changes to the national policies and procedures. Likewise, we receive training in relation to the specific demands and requirements of the FLO co-ordinator role.

How do you manage the potentially conflicting demands of working with service users, colleagues, managers and partners?

As with all parts of the police service there are constant calls on the available duty time. This requires all calls for service to be prioritised. Many members of the public believe that calling 999 will result in the emergency services arriving more quickly than if they call the non-emergency numbers. This is not the case and all calls are assessed, graded and prioritised according to guidelines. In the same way, I prioritise the needs of my 'clients' according to how urgent or life-threatening their issue is or if there are legislative restrictions. The recent floods of 2007 are an example of when the priority of ensuring the safety of the public has to supersede many other responsibilities.

A key to managing these demands is accessibility. By making it clear when I am available ensures that, other than for unexpected high priority demands, I am able to allow the correct amount of time to deal with issues. This also helps me to identify when I need to delegate or seek assistance from colleagues.

In dealing with victims and bereaved families there is a constant balancing act between providing them with the information they want and what has been confirmed.

Case study

While the SIO for a fatal RTC I briefed my FLO on all of the known information for him to pass onto the family. This was done but the uncle of the dead girl, who was the family's point of contact, kept demanding more information. He kept making broad statements about how we knew more and were not telling him. I asked the FLO to explain all that we had confirmed but this was met with a rebuff. Wanting to protect the FLO, as it was her first deployment, I offered to speak with the uncle. Having resolved the initial concerns and fully explained what evidence had been gathered with the greatest sensitivity I thought I had satisfied his needs. However, his calls to the FLO became more frequent. This raised issues as the calls were interfering with her other responsibilities.

In light of this I visited him with the FLO and went through every aspect of the investigation, what evidence had been gathered and what lines of enquiry were still being pursued. I explained how I had been responsible for not allowing access to the scene and the reasons behind my decision, as this had been a continuing complaint. While accepting that progress was being made he kept up some pressure throughout the meeting. However, by spending additional time on this one occasion, I was able to demonstrate that action was being taken and that we were dependent on other agencies for some actions, and was able to reinforce the FLO's position in the investigation.

The regularity of the calls reduced and we maintained a clear line of communication throughout the remainder of the investigation and legal procedures.

Key learning points

- Police officers and police staff use a wide range of interpersonal skills.
- Interactions vary according to the type of incident and person involved.
- Pre-judging a person based on initial information or instincts can lead to adverse reactions by them. Be prepared to amend your viewpoint and your communication methods.
- Interactions can be categorised using Berne's transactional analysis model.
- Betari's box model shows how interactions can be affected by the attitude and displayed behaviour resulting in changes in the attitude and displayed behaviour of the other person in the interaction.
- The feedback sandwich is a useful tool, but it cannot be used as the only method of delivering bad news.

REFLECTION ACTIVITIES

1. One of the challenges of being a police officer is dealing with both victims and perpetrators. What difficulties might this pose for the use of interpersonal skills?
2. Consider how difficult it might be to deliver bad news to the family of someone killed in a RTC. List the skills that might be needed.
3. Watch a television police programme (fictional or documentary), e.g. *The Bill*. Consider how the interactions depicted follow transactional analysis and the Betari's box model. Is there a clear differentiation of rank, role, age, race, gender, etc. in how the interactions are projected?

FURTHER READING

Clements, P. and Jones, J. (2006) *The Diversity Training Handbook: A Practical Guide to Understanding and Changing Attitudes* (2nd ed.). London: Kogan Page

Donnelly, E. and Neville, L. (2008) *Communication and Interpersonal Skills*. Exeter: Reflect Press

Chapter 4

Interpersonal Skills in Welfare Work

Mary Parker

EDITOR'S INTRODUCTION

In this chapter you will read about the work of a welfare officer within the police service. It may increase your understanding of Mary's role if you first read David's chapter on interpersonal skills in the police force. Mary's chapter highlights some of the difficulties that can arise with boundaries when working within a large organisation.

Key themes

- Ethics and confidentiality.
- The importance of supervision.
- Being person-centred.
- Interdisciplinary working.
- Boundaries.

Pre-reading reflection activity

The use of counselling skills is very different from counselling. What do you understand to be the main difference between the two?

MARY PARKER – WELFARE OFFICER

What kind of interactions might you have with people in the course of a normal working day?

I have been working as a welfare officer within the police service for eight years. I gained a Diploma in **Therapeutic Counselling** and, having previously been a police officer, I felt that I could bring knowledge, understanding and empathy to the role.

It may be helpful to understand something of the history in relation to the role of welfare, which is one that exists in organisations such as the Royal Mail and the police, prison, civil and armed services. Welfare provision is constantly changing and responding to the demands of the modern police service. In 1991 the Association of Chief Police Officers instigated a general change in the nature of police welfare work to a concentration on providing support services for serving officers and police staff experiencing a wide range of personal, domestic and work-related problems. Major areas of concern were low morale, high sickness levels and premature retirements. Major national incidents in the 1980s and 1990s, such as Lockerbie in 1988 and Dunblane in 1996, indicated the need for a well-managed and adequately resourced welfare response to support police officers and police staff facing traumatic situations. It has become increasingly important that the work of police welfare providers be part of a co-ordinated and shared approach with, where appropriate, occupational health, health and safety, line management, senior management and staff associations.

What kind of interactions might you have with people in the course of a normal working day?

On a day-to-day basis I work within an Occupational Health, Safety and Welfare Unit, working with managers, personnel staff, police officers, police staff (employees who work within the police service), their families and retired police officers. The client group can raise both work and personal matters, which results in a wide range of potential presenting issues:

- management guidance;
- debt issues;
- relationships;
- change;
- health;
- stress;

- depression;
- grievance;
- housing;
- trauma support.

Sometimes the list seems endless and I still find there are occasions when I am surprised by presenting issues. Referrals come from a variety of sources:

- management;
- self;
- Police Federation;
- UNISON;
- staff associations;
- colleagues.

The majority of individuals that I see are at work and are using welfare support to enable them to stay at work and remain well. I also contribute, in an advisory capacity, to working groups such as 'Ability', which is a staff group advising on disability discrimination issues. The provision of protocols, policies and advice in relation to issues such as stress management, well-being and trauma is also part of my role.

Training and presentations are part of the role for new recruits and sergeants on subjects such as trauma support. One of the more recent provisions within the unit is that of health surveillance where staff, who are identified by managers because of risk assessment in roles such as family liaison, child protection and hostage negotiators, are offered appointments on a one-to-one basis to review their role and discuss how they are managing their own well-being.

Welfare plays an active part in relation to deaths in service, whether that is a death on duty as a result of injury or death off duty. The role is that of a liaison between the family and the organisation to assist the next of kin to deal with funerals, pensions, work issues, dependants and other necessary support. It may also be necessary to undertake some bereavement work with colleagues who may be affected by the death.

One of the most important aspects of a helping relationship is communication. Communication skills 'are not special skills peculiar to helping. Rather they are extensions of the kind of skills all of us need in our everyday interpersonal transactions' (Egan, 1998, p. 90). The ability to communicate effectively in the work place as a welfare officer is not something that is turned on and off for the benefit of clients. It is an integrative way of being. Clients need to experience me in a consistent way.

During the course of a day I would usually work with about four clients on a one-to-one basis either over the phone or face to face. These sessions usually take about one hour. I also deal with enquiries from managers and colleagues, attend meetings and complete written reports and case notes. The stories of Susan and Ryan are examples of the kinds of work that I might do in a typical day.

Case study

Susan exemplifies the type of client who comes for welfare support. She is a police officer in her thirties. A single woman living on her own she joined the police service after a career in the services. Susan has self-referred to Welfare after listening to a presentation about the service on her joining course. She presents as a strong, capable and competent individual who is used to managing on her own. After a few minutes when we have covered the confidentiality contract she breaks down in tears and talks about being embarrassed at the situation she is in financially. Susan explains that she has been spending over a period of months and the trigger for asking for assistance had been that she has been gambling online.

Through the use of counselling skills such as **attending**, listening, **empathy**, focusing and goal setting, Susan agrees to be totally honest about her money circumstances and we work together using clarification and summarising during the session to assess her income, expenditure and total debts. I have a spreadsheet on Excel™ that makes this process easier for both of us as we can see exactly what we are working with. It becomes clear that Susan has a good income with her current wage and a previous employment pension and her outgoings are low. However, she has debt on more than four credit cards, which are now up to their maximum of £7000 per card, a total of £28 000. Every month Susan has kept up at least the minimum payment. However, the interest continues to increase the amount she owes, leaving no margin for living expenses. We go over the options available to her which include:

- family support (i.e. financial or emotional);
- referral to a debt management company for professional financial advice that might include a payment scheme to creditors, an informal voluntary arrangement set up through the county court or bankruptcy.

Some clients come to Welfare at a time in their life when they are in crisis and in these cases listening skills and being empathic is not enough. Advice, guidance and a pragmatic approach may be necessary. This is where welfare work differs from counselling. Susan agrees to the referral and I make the telephone call from the office so that Susan is able to relate her circumstances to the adviser. At the end of the phone conversation I spend some time with Susan using **unconditional positive regard** to work through her choices and her infrastructure of support. We then make arrangements for a follow-up appointment to give her time to consider her options.

At the second appointment Susan seems lighter and is keen to tell me that she has completed the debt management paperwork, her creditors have been contacted and the debt adviser expects the agreement to go ahead without any problems. Susan explains that she has told her family about the debts and, although this was difficult, they are supportive and she no longer feels that she has to financially support them. (Susan had been supporting her family emotionally with 'treats' and did not know how to stop this, especially as she believed that her family saw her as financially secure and successful.)

Since sharing the information about the debts with her family the pressure has been reduced and enabled Susan to concentrate on managing the situation. Susan was embarrassed about the gambling and we talked about her avoidance and the impact it had on her situation. She agreed that when she had sorted out her financial situation she would seek some counselling as she had recognised that the death of one of her parents had been the start of the spending process, a cycle of repeat behaviours and negative automatic thought processes.

Case study

Ryan is a police officer and family liaison officer (FLO) who attends a routine health surveillance appointment for support in relation to the specialist role he undertakes. A FLO would work with bereaved families after a fatal road traffic collision or unusual death. Routine health surveillance addresses well-being, health, sleep, fitness, family, finances and any other issues that could impact on the work–life balance. The session involves listening, using open questions, responding empathically but also challenging in a sensitive appropriate manner. As an operational police officer, the FLO role is an additional responsibility for which he volunteers and for which he has extra training. Ryan currently has two families he is working with and, at the moment, they are both waiting to hear a date for court and inquests.

During the session it becomes clear that over the last few months he has had to deal with some personal issues. His mother in law died suddenly and he has been supporting his wife through her grief. In addition, his young son had been unwell and was undergoing tests at hospital. Ryan did not want to let anyone down. However, he was aware that if anything else occurred he might struggle to cope.

At this point in the session I used the challenge 'I am wondering why you are still taking on FLO roles when you have family health problems?' We reviewed priorities and strategies to manage his role, FLO work was easing up and he agreed to take on no further cases and to identify another FLO who would assist with his families if necessary. In relation to his personal issues he agreed to meet with his manager to discuss the possibility of time off to attend hospital appointments. With this type of collaborative approach it is possible to work with individuals to facilitate an understanding of their own situations and enable them to see things from a different perspective. This in turn enables them to manage a work–life balance and remain well.

In conclusion, Ryan agreed to take on no further FLO work for at least three months and that he would meet with me again before taking on further families. A report to that effect was provided for the FLO manager.

What are the key skills that you use in your work with people?

The toolkit of the welfare officer is extensive. It includes many of the skills learnt through counselling practice:

- listening;
- unconditional positive regard;
- empathy;
- challenge;
- coaching;
- confidentiality;
- goal setting;
- information giving;
- negotiation;
- the ability to create a working alliance with the client.

It is also helpful to have an understanding of the culture of the police service and its working practices, policies and procedures. Within the police service trust is a major issue for staff, therefore the confidentiality of a welfare officer is paramount. I find that clients test the processes around confidentiality; I have a number of clients who have been advised to visit Welfare by colleagues who have experienced and trust the process. The culture of the police service is one of not admitting an inability to cope. Clients might perceive there to be a stigma attached to visiting the welfare officer and, if this is the case, I work with clients to manage their concerns and confidentiality issues.

Counselling is also part of the service I provide. This is agreed with clients in an open and transparent way after assessment, taking into consideration the time available and other options open to the client. We work together to create a verbal contract, which includes the number of sessions and the confidentiality. Elizabeth, Geeta and Ruth are examples of clients who are typical of the sort of day-to-day clients I work with, all of them needing the necessary counselling skills required in the role, although all of them are individual cases with different presenting issues. These case studies demonstrate the versatility and diversity of the welfare officer role.

Case study

Geeta is a young woman, working as a police community support officer (PCSO), who is struggling to manage her work. Geeta has self-referred and presents as a capable, strong-minded woman. Her body language and way of speaking were defensive and my experience of her suggested that she may have a tendency to be confrontational. We complete the assessment process and Geeta told me that she has been diagnosed with dyslexia and attention deficit disorder. Geeta presents very competently and articulates very well. However, she struggles to read large amounts of text and cannot concentrate on written work. Therefore she is constantly behind with work and stuck in a negative cycle of not being able to get paperwork in on time.

Geeta: I get frustrated when I am asked to read large documents.
Me: Is there anything that might ease that pressure? [open question].
Geeta: More time I guess.
Me: I wonder what would have to happen for you to get more time?
Geeta: I could ask the Sergeant.

As a practitioner I believe that assessment is an important part of the process and, in this case, I found that not all **cognitive behavioural therapy** (CBT) techniques such as, for example, written homework are suitable for some clients and I have found it necessary to adapt the process for clients with learning issues.

In counselling sessions I would routinely ask clients to keep thought diaries based on their negative automatic thought processes. In this case, however, I sensed that Geeta would not continue with the work if it was perceived in any way 'too difficult'. However, Geeta did work with her thought processes well, and when I drew them on paper and shared with her, she was easily able to recognise patterns. For example, she could see that her trigger would be something like being asked to break the vicious circles that I drew as she talked.

Trigger: Asked to read a complex portfolio. This led her to a negative thought that she wouldn't understand it, which made her feel anxious and embarrassed. She then avoided doing the work creating the vicious circle of always being late with her paperwork.

Negative thought: I won't understand.
Emotion: Anxious, embarrassed.
Behaviour: Walks away – avoids.

Geeta worked hard to change her thought processes and reported that she felt less angry. At the end of her sessions with me I referred Geeta to a mentoring programme, working with her to select a mentor suitable to empower her to change issues for herself and to find ways of working smarter with paperwork.

Case study

Elizabeth is a member of police staff and a manager. She has been off work sick for about eight weeks and has self-referred on the advice of a friend. I visited Elizabeth at home and found that she was concerned about her health and awaiting appointments and tests at the hospital. Her GP had referred her to the community psychiatric nurse (CPN). Elizabeth was presenting with anxiety, which was having such an impact on her that she was only leaving the house to attend medical appointments or to visit close friends. The anxiety was based around her intellectual abilities and an overwhelming fear that she could be perceived as stupid and incapable.

In the first couple of sessions I worked to build the relationship and an understanding of her thought processes. I also lent her Elizabeth Padesky and Greenberger's *Mind Over Mood* (see the Further Reading list at the end of this chapter) which had been prescribed by her CPN. Cognitive techniques were discussed relating to how to balance thinking and challenge negative automatic thought processes. I also did some work with Elizabeth to identify coping strategies to balance out any rumination such as daily walks, cooking and engaging with friends. An appointment was made for Elizabeth to see the occupational health doctor at her place of work but this was something that she was unable to consider. It was not talking to the doctor that caused her concern

▶

but going into the workplace and the possibility of meeting colleagues. The fear was very real and the anxiety so intense it evoked thoughts of suicide. Elizabeth's refusal to attend the appointment, even though she offered to meet at an alternative venue, have a home visit or talk on the phone, was perceived by her manager and occupational health staff as her being difficult.

The clients that I see are not always presenting as they do in their day-to-day work environment. I sometimes observe glimpses of the real person behind the facade. Most of the time Elizabeth presented as a confident, capable woman who was very articulate. It was only on peeling back the layers that it was possible to see a very insecure, scared child. It is likely that Elizabeth's manager could not see beyond the presenting image and was unable to understand why Elizabeth could not return to the workplace.

Hospital tests were completed and the diagnosis identified that the health problems could be managed by diet. This obviously lifted a huge weight of concern from Elizabeth and although there was an improvement in her anxiety it was not a magic cure.

Elizabeth is working on returning to the workplace, challenging negative thoughts and anxieties, developing coping strategies and creating an infrastructure of people that she can seek out for support if she needs it.

Case study

Ruth is a police widow. Her husband died in 1957 in an accident on duty while he was riding a police motorcycle. I have routine contact with Ruth in relation to support from the Police Dependants' Trust, which provides financial support for dependants of officers who are killed or injured on duty. Ruth's daughter contacted me and asked if I could visit her mum about her current situation. I called at Ruth's home, a three-bedroom family house, which she keeps in a very neat condition. Ruth has been unwell with an ongoing condition but she has also recently fallen down the stairs and broken her arm. This has reinforced a need to move to a smaller home while she is still well enough to manage the situation. I talked through the options with Ruth and her daughter, who lives nearby. Sometimes listening to the client is not enough but, as in Ruth's case, practical help can facilitate effective life changes.

Ruth would like to remain living in the same area to maintain her infrastructure of existing support. The difficulty is that bungalows in the area are valued at the same amount as her own home but she has insufficient savings to pay the cost of the move such as, for example, removal, solicitors and estate agents. I helped her to make an application to the Police Dependants' Trust for assistance and they were able to finance the cost of the move. Ruth moved into a small bungalow a couple of streets away, in the same community, therefore extending the time that she will be able to spend in her own home.

What is the legislative framework which underpins your practice?

Legislation, particularly the Health and Safety at Work Act 1974 and the Police (Health and Safety) Act 1997, prompted police forces to assess the nature and scale of risk to health in the workplace for both police officers and police staff and to devise procedures to address such issues. This legislation is therefore central to my practice.

In respect of the Children's Acts 1989 and 2004 and child protection legislation issues I work within the British Association of Counselling and Psychotherapy (BACP) Ethical Framework and, if a child protection issue is raised by a client and I need to breach confidentiality, initially I would take advice from my clinical supervisor and or the head of the Police Child Protection Team.

In addition it is important for me to have a working knowledge of Police Regulations, which govern police officers' terms and conditions of service, pensions regulations and benefits advice.

What theoretical models underpin your practice?

My counselling qualification is a Therapeutic Counselling Diploma. The model I use most with clients is based in **cognitive behavioural therapy (CBT)**, which identifies feelings, patterns of behaviour and negative automatic thought processes and considers evidence to support the change of the thought processes. It is a practical model. Cognitive behavioural therapy examines the client's reality testing system. It encourages exchange of information, works within a collaborative approach and teaches clients how to evaluate and modify thinking while focusing on symptom relief and developing adaptive behaviours. The timeframe for more time-consuming therapies in the workplace is restricted and the practical, shorter approach of CBT enables them to continue personal development after the sessions have concluded.

> Compared to antidepressants, CBT is as effective in the short term and more effective in the long term in the treatment of mild and moderate depression and anxiety disorders. It reduces the symptoms of the illness and prevents them from returning. CBT has also been found to be effective in helping people stay in their jobs when they become unwell with depression. (Seymour and Grove, 2008)

What are the ethical issues that impact on your practice?

As a counsellor and welfare officer I am professionally governed by two codes of ethics that include guidance on my working practice.

1. The British Association of Counselling and Psychotherapy Ethical Framework:

   BACP Ethics for Counselling and Psychotherapy unifies and replaces all the earlier codes for counsellors, trainers and supervisors and is also applicable to counselling research, the use of counselling skills and the management of these services within organisations. It is intended to inform the practice of each member of the British Association for Counselling and Psychotherapy. (BACP, 2007)

2. National Association of Welfare Advisers' (NAPWA) Values, Principles and Moral Qualities:

   All clients are entitled to good standards of practice and care from their Police Welfare Service. Good standards of practice and care require professional competence; good relationships with clients and colleagues; and commitment to and observance of professional ethics. (NAPWA, 2007)

Joe is an example of a client with whom I had to pay particular attention to my code of ethics.

Case study

Joe has been referred to me by his manager who is concerned about his well-being and specifically about his relationship with his wife. Joe has a poor attendance record and has recently reported to work with injuries, in particular scratches on his face.

Joe is in his early twenties and has been a police officer for two years. He has two children under two years old. His wife is 18 and they have been living together for several years. I explain the confidentiality of the session, which was that it might be necessary for me to breach confidentiality in respect of terrorism, child protection or if there is the possibility of harm to another. Joe explains that he has told his sergeant about his situation and that his wife has hit him on several occasions. She likes to go out to nightclubs and gets angry if he is working and there is no babysitter or if he mentions about her drinking. Joe makes it quite clear that he has talked to his supervisor and that at no time has he physically hurt his wife and that he does not want to take any formal action about her behaviour.

I work with Joe to review how he wants to spend the time with me. He chooses to use the session to review how he is going to care for his family and the pressure to manage a full-time job role while worrying about the family. During the session Joe mentioned that a neighbour approached him because she had seen his wife smacking the little boy in the garden. He did not know how to manage the situation. In summarising what Joe had told me I was able to clarify my understanding of what had been disclosed and this enabled me to consider a serious practitioner dilemma, which was that the children might be at risk. In this situation I needed to follow my professional codes of conduct. These required that I put the safety of children before my contract with my client.

Consequently, as I had explained to Joe about the limitations of the confidentiality between us at the beginning, I was now able to explain about the child protection issues and talk about the options with him:

- that Joe tells his line manager about the situation with me;
- that I discuss the situation with my clinical supervisor to review whether it is necessary to breach confidentiality and to whom;

►

- that I contact the BACP legal helpline for advice as to the way forward;
- with Joe's permission, I tell the Child Protection Unit supervisor;
- Joe and I together seek advice from the Child Protection Unit supervisor.

Joe agreed to invite a member of the Child Protection Team to join us and he then repeated the story told by his neighbour. Recommendations were made by the officer to discreetly notify the social services department and arrange for a home visit to be made, without identifying the source of the information to protect the neighbour. It is important to use supervision in cases of confidentiality or disclosure as it is not always necessary for the therapist to breach the confidentiality. When working within a clear ethical framework and contract with the client, individuals can be empowered to manage the ethical issues for themselves.

In follow-up sessions I worked with Joe while he considered the options available to him. A network of family and additional support was put in place and, some months later, Joe's wife left the family, leaving the children with their father.

Working with people can be very demanding. How do you care for yourself?

I see a clinical supervisor for one and half hours every month in line with the BACP recommendations. He works with a cognitive behavioural therapy model focusing on case formulation, which I find very helpful. He is challenging, especially around the boundaries between welfare and counselling work. I have also found that he is adaptable and if I need to explore relationships in the workplace that I find are impacting on my work such as, for example when I have felt unsupported by my line management, he is able to help me to focus on the processes and enables me to balance out my thought processes. If I feel it necessary I will seek additional supervision sessions to enable me to manage personal issues at work that could impact on my professional practice.

Working with Trauma Support is one area of my work where I find clinical supervision invaluable. It is important for me to acknowledge what I hear from my clients and yet, with this support, I can separate myself from the actual event and the possibility of secondary trauma.

Case study

Cilla is a control room operator who has been referred by her line manager for Trauma Support. Cilla is in her forties and she has considerable experience in the role, having worked in the control room for over ten years. This role involves taking calls from members of the public, including 999 emergency calls, recording the information on the computer and allocating officers to attend incidents. Cilla has taken a 999 call from a woman who was being attacked by her ex-partner with a knife.

A Trauma Support meeting has a clear structure:

- talking about the facts of the situation;
- clarifying how staff are feeling;
- giving educative advice on how trauma can affect individuals;
- giving details of the available support network.

Facts

Cilla has taken the call from a woman who is very scared and it has been difficult to get her to talk because the ex-partner is shouting in the background and there are thumping noises. Cilla deploys officers to the scene and continues to talk to the woman while colleagues assist with the management of the incident. Initially the conversation was difficult because of the noise in the background, then the man leaves the room and the woman is on her own. However, she seems dazed and Cilla is unable to get very much conversation before she hears a choking noise and the line is cut off.

Feelings

Cilla was shocked to learn that the woman had died of stab wounds; she is upset and angry. Cilla talked about the waste of a life and feeling disempowered because she could not get medical help to the woman sooner. It was recognised that the nature of the attack was violent and also that Cilla would not change how she had dealt with the incident. Cilla also acknowledged that, although she was not there in person to assist, she had been able

▶

---

to talk on the telephone to the woman and was hopeful that this may have given the woman some comfort.

Future

We discussed practical issues such as the impact of adrenaline after the incident, whether Cilla was sleeping normally, her available support network and strategies for coping and distracting herself from distressing thoughts and images.

A follow-up meeting was arranged for one month after this meeting and Cilla, although still sad about the loss of life, had the incident in perspective and therefore required no further support.

Trauma Support work fits well within the Mearns and Dryden (1990) view of counselling: 'Counselling is like living with your finger on the fast forward button; you can go through an enormous amount of living in just one hour.' However, it is important, as a practitioner working with trauma and listening to potentially distressing events, to keep things in perspective; this is the client's experience, not mine, and to maintain my own well-being I need to keep them separate.

How do you ensure that your practice responds to current research?

As a member of the British Association of Counselling and Psychotherapy I am constantly made aware of the current issues within counselling through the monthly *Therapy* magazine.

I am a member of the National Association of Police Welfare Advisers and have been the National Secretary for the past two years. This association meets on a quarterly basis, usually in London, and we discuss current issues, provide support to members on ethical matters and provide training for both new welfare officers and existing members. There is a National Training Conference once a year. Last year the theme of the conference was 'Psychological Preparedness in the Police Service'. Training like this not only provides education on current practices for us but also provides techniques and information that we can pass on to clients. The conference also provides an opportunity to network with colleagues. The world of Police Welfare is a small one and meeting colleagues and having an insight into their work is always beneficial. The value of having an opportunity to wind down with friends and colleagues should not be underestimated.

How are your continuing professional development needs fulfilled?

The NAPWA annual training conference provides opportunities for continuous professional development hours. Debt management companies and agencies such as the Child Support Agency regularly provide training updates. In recent years I have attended short courses on subjects such as Trauma Management and Coaching. To widen my CPD opportunities, outside my daily working environment, I have also participated in training and tutoring at a further education college on the Counselling Diploma Course. Currently, I am providing clinical supervision for four diploma students in a group session. I find that this allows me to develop outside of my day-to-day role of welfare and work from a different perspective, creating some personal and professional balance.

How do you manage the potentially conflicting demands of working with service users, colleagues, managers and partners?

I have developed an infrastructure of support through colleagues, peer groups and counselling to manage the conflicts and issues that are sometimes raised within the welfare role. The most difficult aspect of my role is working with other health professionals who have a different code of ethics, specifically regarding confidentiality, and managing their expectations of information in relation to clients. My experience is that medical confidentiality is very different to that of the welfare and counselling codes of practice and, although I accept that working collaboratively can be very effective, it should not be done at the cost of the client's confidentiality and trust.

Trust is central to my work with clients and I endorse the personal moral qualities (BACP, 2007) for the use of counselling skills in the workplace. These qualities have also been adopted by NAPWA. They are available at **www.bacp.co.uk/admin/structure/files/pdf/ethical_framework_web.pdf**.

Key learning points

- Welfare work is very different from counselling. It does involve some of the same skills, but counselling does not include the giving of advice.
- Supervision and the support of others are vital for maintaining personal well-being in both counselling and welfare work.
- There can be conflicts between different professionals in the same setting.
- Techniques may have to be adapted to suit individuals' specific needs.
- The ability to communicate effectively in the workplace as a welfare officer is not something that is turned on and off for the benefit of clients.

REFLECTION ACTIVITIES

1. Think of a role or a situation that you have experienced where you have used or could have used counselling skills. What skills do you think you used?
2. What do you think are the most important skills for a welfare officer to have?
3. Reflect on what you believe would be the most important skills to have as a welfare officer in the police service?
3. If you were employed within the police service what provision would you expect from the welfare officer?

FURTHER READING

Aldridge, S. and Rigby, S. (2001) *Counselling Skills in Context*. Rugby: Hodder & Stoughton and BACP

Culley, S. and Bond, T. (2004) *Integrative Counselling Skills in Action*. London: Sage

Padesky, C. and Greenberger, D. (1995) *Mind Over Mood: Change How You Feel By Changing the Way You Think*. London: Guilford Press

Chapter 5

Interpersonal Skills in Community Social Work

Joy Gauci

EDITOR'S INTRODUCTION

'Social workers form partnerships with people, helping them to assess and interpret the problems they face, and supporting them in finding solutions' (DoH, 2008). These partnerships necessitate the development of effective interpersonal skills. Seden (2005) suggests that in social work the social worker and service user have not usually chosen to be in a relationship with each other and that this may create an initial barrier. This highlights the importance of forming and sustaining relationships through effective interpersonal skills.

In this chapter you will read about Joy's work as a community social worker attached to a community health centre operating within the Primary Care Trust.

Key themes

- Diversity.
- Vulnerability.
- Marginalisation.
- Evidence-based practice.
- Supervision.

Pre-reading reflection activity

Go to **www.socialworkcareers.co.uk/socialwork/what/meet. asp** and read about the work and cases of social workers in different settings. In each role you will be able to identify key interpersonal skills.

JOY GAUCI – COMMUNITY SOCIAL WORKER

The function of contemporary social work is ever changing as it reacts to societal change and political drivers. It is a profession with a traditional association of providing welfare support for people who are vulnerable and representing marginalised groups (see the section on page 87 on legal frameworks). Social work also has an interest in community action: striving to promote diversity and minority rights for individuals who may not be members of legally defined vulnerable groups, but who might still require particular support at times of need or transition.

In this chapter, I will explore how I have worked with a range of people, predominantly in partnership with people from traditional groups of **vulnerable adults**, including adults with physical disabilities, learning difficulties, mental health needs and dementia. My work also included working in partnership and providing support for informal carers.

I will consider my work with individuals at stages of transition, need or crisis, exploring the way that theoretical frameworks guided my interventions to nurture positive changes.

Describe the kind of interactions you would have with people in the course of a normal working day

Healy (2005) suggests the primary roles of the social worker include risk management, implementation of statutory law, support and advocacy, therapeutic intervention, community education and community action. As a specialist social worker in a community health team, I was expected to undertake a range of administrative, procedural and more therapeutic roles, including the following key roles and duties.

Statutory social work duties

A statutory social worker has a legal responsibility to undertake assessments for children and vulnerable adults who are either in need of support or 'at risk' of abuse or neglect. The Children Act 1989 provides the mandate for responses to children at risk of 'significant harm' (section 47), and also identifies key responsibilities for children with particular needs. The NHS and Community Care Act 1990 identifies the duty to assess (section 47) adults deemed vulnerable and in potential need of support services. *No Secrets* (DoH, 2000) provides guidance rather than legal mandate, but has emphasised the social work responsibility to intervene to protect vulnerable adults at risk, again, of 'significant harm'.

Significant harm is consequently the baseline for intervening to protect either vulnerable children or adults.

I am a specialist social worker for vulnerable adults so I undertake all the legal duties with vulnerable adults outlined above. This involves making assessments of vulnerable adults at points of transition or when exposed to a risk. I am not an approved social worker or specialist child protection worker, hence I would screen any referrals to be passed on to the relevant child protection, family support and specialist mental health teams.

Partnership working

Responsibility to assess, monitor and review translates into a working partnership traditionally described as 'case work' (Biestek, 1957). It has **humanistic** origins, based on the idea of the care giver working with the individual over a period of time to enable the exploration of feelings and to create frameworks for responses to the needs identified. The humanistic belief in the individual's capacity for growth and development, for 'self-actualisation' (Howe, 1987), underpins the value basis of the relationship. While there is recognition that the relationship should have a balance based on equal respect, there needs to be an acknowledgement that there are inevitable power differentials between the care receiver and care giver. The power base of the relationship has been explored particularly over the last ten years (Dominelli, 2002; Thompson, 2005), echoing the increasing recognition of active citizenship rights for vulnerable people.

The majority of my interactions would fall into this category of case or partnership working with vulnerable adults. In addition, I also work in partnership with informal carers to support them in sustaining long-term caring relationships with vulnerable adults living in the community. I have a legal duty identified in the Carers (Recognition and Services) Act 1995 to provide informal carers with an assessment.

Gatekeeper, signposter and advocate

The therapeutic aspects of the helping relationship are described above. If specific needs are identified in the working partnership, the social worker has a responsibility to liaise or network to provide resources and other support services. The social worker acts as gatekeeper to social services or contracted services provided by private and voluntary sector welfare.

The social worker also has a signposting role to provide the service user with information about support services and resources across the range of social work, community health, voluntary and private welfare and more general community and neighbourhood services. This role works particularly well when a social worker operates from a GP surgery, as people calling to access community health services can receive information about social work and broader community resources at the same time.

Liaising for services and resources for vulnerable and marginalised adults can require an advocative role to ensure their rights are promoted and protected. Advocacy in social work has a dual expectation:

- to ensure all sections of the community have equal access to services;
- to ensure that historically disadvantaged individuals and groups (who may not have legal associations of vulnerability) whether because they are homeless, have a drug or alcohol dependency or a range of other factors, still have their full citizenship rights promoted.

This is also a natural role for the social worker in a GP surgery, as all sectors of the community are represented in this context, including marginalised groups.

Examples of interventions in my work (using the roles identified above)

- Assessment and support for an individual at the point of diagnosis of a physical disability.
- Supporting a relative who is caring for someone with a terminal illness.
- Identifying needs and planning resource support for an individual transferring home from hospital.
- Intervening to support an individual at a point of crisis at home, for example after sustaining a fall, or when a main carer has been admitted to hospital.
- Signposting for a young person who has left foster care.
- Providing resources for individuals, e.g. **respite care**, rehabilitative day care, personal care support at home.
- Assessment – to support and monitor a vulnerable adult like, for example, an older woman with dementia or a younger man with acquired brain injury, to enable them to sustain independent living in the community.
- Interacting to safeguard a vulnerable adult at risk of 'significant harm' in the form of neglect, abuse or hardship.

What are the key skills that you use in your work with people?

The specific duty of the social worker to respond to individuals at points of need or transition has been identified. This is an exacting requirement which requires theory and knowledge to be used in a particular way. The range of roles, duties and skills of the social worker has also been identified. Consequently, social work, as a profession, needs a knowledge base that promotes responsiveness to the individual by providing a range of theories. The tension is in responding to the individual in a flexible, valuing way, but also within an objective, evidence-based framework. This has been described as the tension between the 'technical rational', which focuses on outcomes and evidence, and the 'professional artist', characterised by holistic, **experiential** approaches to learning (Fish and Coles, 2005).

I would suggest that the social worker is trained to be skilled to draw on traditions of both science and art – in actual fact to draw a baseline of knowledge to form an objective critical axis, combined with a dynamic responsiveness to the experience of the individual in their particular context. This responsiveness has a subjective element based on respect for the individual, their view of their experience and their capacity to draw on their own resourcefulness and insight to move through the experience. The **reflexive** sensitivity of the social worker allows him or her to recognise the impact of 'use of self' – the worker's identity, values and skills and the way these also influence the working relationship.

Finally, the social worker draws on skills of reflective practice to evaluate the value and quality of the interaction, to learn from the experience and plan the next part of the process. This promotes 'experiential learning' (Kolb, 1984) where the social worker creates knowledge based on professional experience. This is often termed practice wisdom.

Specific uses of knowledge in social work practice

Payne (2005) identifies a hierarchy of knowledge the social worker needs to draw on:

1. **To understand the world**. Formal knowledge traditions create a framework for objective critical analysis like, for example, functionalism, Marxism, liberalism. These provide a framework in which to understand and respond to human need.

2. **To underpin specific approaches to interventions**. A range of approaches based on traditions from psychology, philosophy and sociology forms the methods of social work interventions such as, for example, partnership working, task-centred working, crisis interventions, use of counselling skills.

I would add a third category of knowledge usage:

3. **Knowledge and understanding of reflective, reflexive and experiential knowledge**. Models of reflective and reflexive practice promote critical awareness of 'use of self' and critical analysis of the quality of an individual's interactions.

This complex balance, drawing on various components of the relationship working, is, arguably, the trademark of social work as a profession. It is a profession that promotes a reflective climate recognising that the knowledge drawn from interactions with vulnerable and **marginalised people** is as valid as traditions of formal knowledge. This consequently promotes the voice of marginalised groups and nurtures radical and alternative perspectives to challenge structural hierarchy and the status quo. This has allowed social work practice to embrace the liberation movements of feminism, disability activism, anti-racism and gay liberation, for example, with their challenge of knowledge elitism.

Case study

Bayo is a 48-year-old black South African man married to Ellen, a 42-year-old English woman. They have a son aged 14. Ellen and her son have been staying with Ellen's mother because of complex marital circumstances resulting from the care scenario. Bayo has had ME for four years and has been unable to work. He has variable but often considerably restricted mobility so tends to live downstairs in their home. He has also had clinical depression for 18 months. Ellen has been working part-time and caring for Bayo, but their relationship has become strained to a point where Ellen feels the demands on her are too great. She wants the marriage to continue, but does not see how the tension will be resolved. Bayo feels it is her duty as his wife to provide for his care needs and is reluctant to discuss the issues between them.

Bayo's GP has requested that the social worker visit to talk with Bayo and Ellen, particularly focusing on their financial concerns and Bayo's recreational and personal care needs, but also to be sensitive to the fact that they might request advice about seeking marital support. When the social worker visits, Bayo suggests Ellen retreat to the kitchen while he discusses his support needs with the social worker. He has prepared for the assessment visit and plans to focus on his health, personal care, financial and recreational needs.

This situation involves complex dynamics. Bayo needs support as he struggles emotionally and physically to manage a condition that has long-term implications and which is currently rendering an active, resourceful man largely housebound. However, he is viewing his needs in isolation and failing to recognise their impact on his wife and son. Ellen is struggling emotionally to continue holding main carer responsibility in a marriage in which the dynamics have radically changed; Bayo is reluctant to acknowledge these tensions and assumes it is his wife's duty to perform this role. Ellen is also main carer for their son, Matthew, undertakes part-time work and provides all domestic support as well as some physical care tasks for Bayo on days when his condition requires this. There is an additional tension created by cultural expectations of gender and role.

Matthew is currently staying with his grandmother, resentful of the change in family life and trying to negate his emotional needs with a buoyant social life.

The social worker has to decide how to respond to the competing needs of Bayo and Ellen, recognising the potential conflict of interest and making a value judgement about the appropriateness of focusing on Bayo's needs as he expects (technically he is the service user), hence potentially colluding with the marginalisation of Ellen. The social worker has a professional responsibility to promote anti-oppressive and anti-racist practice; yet supporting Bayo's cultural identity could potentially create oppression for Ellen as the situation suggests gender and role stereotyping have occurred.

▶

Use of theory:

To understand the situation

1. Recognition of structural causes of marginalisation, in particular relating to culture, disability and gender identity and function.
2. Philosophical theory to consider the value of respect for persons and promote individual responses that will allow each party support for their rights.
3. Understanding of psychological and human developmental theories to understand how people react and find support in complex human situations.

These theories can help the worker identify the needs of all three individuals in the family:

- Bayo, who experiences loss of physical health, physical independence and social and recreational activity;
- Ellen, who recognises the change in relationship and family dynamics and reacts to the overwhelming burden of responsibility;
- Matthew, who is at a stage of transition between child and adulthood and has his own emotional and psychological needs at a time when the priority focus is on his father's ill health and the consequent marital tension.

To form a plan of intervention

The social worker draws on a range of methods and tools developed in social work practice in her intervention. There are options:

- work with the family as a unit, or the couple as a unit, drawing on systems theory and using techniques from family and relationship therapy;
- work with each family member individually, using techniques from partnership working to create a trust-based relationship in which to explore need and using counselling techniques to allow insight and reframing and drawing on individual resources to create change.

If the second of these plans is undertaken, it may require two workers, working separately with Bayo and Ellen, should the tensions created by the conflict of interest risk worker collusion. Matthew might need an advocate in his own right.

To critically evaluate the professional intervention

An awareness of reflective and reflexive practice allows me to recognise and evaluate the impact of personal values and professional identity on my understanding of, and responsiveness to, the situation. The following model of reflective questions can be used to evaluate both the use of self and the outcome of the intervention:

- What am I trying to do in this interaction?
- What are my basic assumptions about this situation?
- How will these assumptions affect the way I work?
- What approaches am I going to use?
- How will I check if these approaches have worked?

(Redmond, 2006)

What is the legislative framework that underpins your practice?

The legislative framework that underpins my role as a social worker is discussed in depth throughout the text. Applicable legislation includes:

Carers (Recognition and Services) Act 1995;
NHS and Community Care Act 1990;
Children Act 1989;
Children Act 2004;
Human Rights Act 1998;
Disability Discrimination Act 1986.

What are the key communication skills that you use in your work with people?

The case study demonstrates three fundamental requirements of good social work practice:

- skills to engage in critical thinking;
- skills to communicate and engage in partnership working with vulnerable or marginalised people;
- skills to be able to advocate and negotiate at points of conflict.

In my relationship work, Seden's model of surface and depth communication has been valid. It suggests the social worker draws on skills of initial exchange to build understanding and create rapport between the care giver and care receiver. It also promotes active listening, hence allows for responsiveness to individuality of experience. It is essential in the case study to recognise the different ways that Bayo, Ellen and Matthew have all reacted to Bayo's health crisis and resultant change of identity and role. Validating their individual experiences can allow for the development of a relationship of trust.

The assessment procedure may be hindered by the service user or carer's overwhelming sense of grief, frustration, anger or fear. Seden identifies the use of counselling skills at such times to allow a deeper expression of feeling. The worker's skills of active listening and responsiveness potentially allow the individual to explore their personal experience on a level of depth. Bayo, for example, might choose to explore his emotional needs – the reaction to his ill health, the impact on his personal relationships and social life, his concerns about the future.

Communication at a depth level draws on a range of counselling skills, including ventilation of feelings, active listening, prompting, clarifying, removing blocks, understanding defences and reactions to loss, and reframing (Seden, 2005).

Finally, there is a distinctive use of therapeutic skills in social work practice to promote the value base of social work. This is deeper than a respect for difference and diversity of experience. It is the recognition of the responsibility of the worker to engender a sense of service user confidence and self-belief. This is promoted in the partnership relationship, where the worker in the case study can allow Bayo to explore aspects of his identity, including his cultural background and his life experience.

What theoretical models underpin your practice?

I use a range of theoretical models in my interventions with people. The reflective model has already been considered. A critical understanding of the professional use of self can be promoted using a model based on the concept of emotional intelligence (Salovey and Mayer, cited in Howe, 2008):

- the perception and expression of emotion in the self and others;
- the use of emotion to facilitate thought;
- understanding and analysing emotions in self and others;
- regulating and managing emotions in self and others depending on one's needs, goals and plans (the management of relationships).

In addition, I would particularly promote a model of anti-oppression and an empowerment-based model of intervention. Thompson's (2005) anti-oppressive model considers the three strands of oppression – personal, cultural and structural. This model allows me to identify the potential barriers a person might experience in their identity as a service user, and to focus on the restrictions these might cause to the individual.

The 'strengths perspective' attributed to Reynolds (1951) has an empowerment basis to its approach. Healy suggests this approach changes the way that we listen and respond to the person's narrative, heightening a sensitivity to recognise the person's capacity for growth and resourcefulness. This is a challenge to too dominant a focus on vulnerability and risk.

1. Adopt an optimistic attitude.
2. Focus primarily on assets.
3. Collaborate with the service user.
4. Work towards the long-term empowerment of service users.
5. Create community.

(Healy, 2005)

This model is particularly suited to casework practice in social work as it emphasises the importance of social identity and interdependency.

What are the ethical issues that impact on your practice?

The British Association for Social Work (BASW) Code of Ethics (2002) identifies the broad principles of the value framework in which social workers operate, promoting:

- human dignity and worth;
- social justice;
- service to humanity;
- integrity;
- competence.

These are based on the idea or vision of the social worker as the agent of social justice. These principles provide a valid and action-guiding baseline for the partnership working, reminding the social worker of their role to nurture the individual's sense of identity and capacity for growth. The concept of service to humanity reminds the social worker that the relationship develops in a societal context rather than in isolation – a reminder that the social worker may need to promote the rights of the individual to protect social justice!

There is a tension, however, between the social worker as agent of social justice and the social work role as agent of the state. This can result in value tensions – to promote social justice in a climate of resource restrictions, to promote empowerment but also to have, at times, to restrain an individual who is at risk of harm.

Working with people can be very demanding. How do you care for yourself?

One of the great motivators for me in being able to work with individuals on such a personal level is the value of this individual sense of connectedness and potential empathy. However, it is important to be clear about the role we undertake in our practice, and to protect the boundaries of that role. This is a complex balance in social work where we often request the sharing of deeply personal information and experience on the part of the service user or carer. Social workers often talk of the professional responsibility to give back to the individual a sense of themselves and their own identity. This is a complex balance, however, because it is also essential to retain a more neutral objectivity.

It is fundamentally an idealistic notion to respond to need and create positive change and I do recognise the need to retain a sense of realism in my practice. Models of supervision in the social work profession allow a protected space for reflection on personal well-being as well as accountable professional practice. This conveys a message about their intrinsic connectedness. I believe we have a responsibility to clients and colleagues to be critically in touch with our own sense of physical, emotional and spiritual well-being. I do not feel I could assume that social work is a profession for life as I recognise that there might be periods in my own life when I might not have the emotional resilience to sustain support for others.

Some social workers sustain their motivation and reflective practice by changing team or the context of their social work. I have had opportunities to do this – to work in different contexts of practice with different client groups and to work in different areas of the UK – which I have found to be personally helpful. I also had a period of time out of social work practice and undertook a piece of research to allow me to return to practice feeling better informed and refreshed.

How do you ensure your practice responds to current research?

I value the current emphasis on evidence-informed practice that draws from formal sources of knowledge and orthodox research. The study that I undertook was an evaluation of the research highlighting the prevalence of vulnerable adult abuse and neglect in particular contexts of welfare practice. This research springboarded the White Paper, *No Secrets* (DoH, 2000), promoting the responsibility to safeguard the protective rights of vulnerable adults. I returned to social work practice with a clearer awareness both of the prevalence of the issue and the responsibility of the social worker to identify and challenge oppressive practice. I valued the framework of *No Secrets* in giving a proactive guide to safeguard vulnerable adults at risk of abuse or neglect.

I also recognise the value of empirical research for social work practice. The interesting aspect of the strengths approach discussed on page 89 was that it was based on empirical research about psychological resilience. Saleebey's review of research (cited in Healy, 2005) noted the psychological strength of children experiencing childhood trauma and adversity. This is invaluable research in promoting welfare practice which emphasises resourcefulness as a potential challenge to the traditional welfare emphasis on vulnerability.

Social work as a profession values action research – drawing on the service user experience to promote marginalised voices and hence to challenge orthodoxy of opinion. The work of the Social Care Institute for Excellence (SCIE) promotes front-line knowledge that allows for diverse perspectives in learning. Research projects based on framing and questioning to present a variety of possibilities rather than a problem-solving approach are particularly valid as they develop attitudes that difference is acceptable. This message is linked to the notion of equal citizenship rights.

How are your continuing professional development needs fulfilled?

I would view my journey of CPD as a relationship between reflective learning (the student journey) and reflective practice (the qualified social work path). I believe there is a risk that the establishment of a reflective climate developed in the higher education institution (HEI) becomes narrower in a practice setting if too strong a focus is placed on outcomes and targets. While a clear sense of direction and organisational accountability is important, target- and competency-based approaches can risk the promotion of technical knowledge and proficiency over a sustained questioning and reflective stance.

The social worker needs to be able to sustain motivation to learn and reflect. My personal technique for protecting this balance was to qualify as a practice assessor to provide practice-based learning opportunities for social workers in training (initially for the Diploma in Social Work then latterly for the degree). This allowed me to keep up to date with social work education, to challenge and reflect on my own social work practice, and to promote a culture of dialogue and reflective learning in my social work team.

I am currently employed as a lecturer in social work education, but combine this role with practice and research to protect my CPD.

How do you manage the conflicting demands of working with service users, colleagues and managers?

Work with service users

I expect my work with service users and carers to be challenging and emotionally charged. This can appear daunting in abstract but the negative emotions that a service user might have – distress, anxiety and anger – can also be counterbalanced in practice realities with glimpses of unreserved humour, resourcefulness and insight. There is often a true and moving sense of sharing the richness of human experience. This has struck me often after reading a referral requesting an assessment visit where I have had a sense of the individual's overwhelming need or vulnerability. When visiting the individual, however, I have seen not a frail, dependent person but a dignified, resilient and resourceful individual. The isolated (and disabled) older farmer cheerfully describing to me how he used the foot of his Zimmer frame to punch holes in the soil for his seed potatoes is a good example! I was struck by his resourcefulness rather than his isolation and disability.

Realistically, of course, the opposite can occur when you respond to a seemingly 'routine' referral to find the main carer has had a stroke or the disabled adult has sustained a fall hence requiring a complex balance of support needs. In such scenarios, it is important to recognise the complexity, find space for reflection with a colleague or supervisor, and compose a clear plan of action recognising role, boundary of role and competing tensions. It is particularly complex responding to a crisis or trauma if your work culture only allows a single assessment visit. One of the strengths of the assessment model promoted in the NHS Community Care Act 1990 is that it promotes a sustained working relationship or 'partnership' with the service user as you move through the process of assessment, monitoring and review. This process allows for reflection and revisit so that any sense of work that was incomplete or unpursued in an earlier visit due to charged emotion or conflict can be regained.

Work with colleagues

In a community health setting, I worked as closely with colleagues from community health as with fellow social workers. I also worked closely with colleagues in the private and voluntary sector including housing wardens and day centre and rehabilitation unit workers. There were occasions when there were tensions between professional perspectives stemming out of the medical and social models of welfare practice, as my health colleagues had a responsibility to identify and protect against medical risk whereas the culture of social work intrinsically promotes choice, autonomy and individual responsibility in life choices. It is too linear to suggest that community health promotes only the medical model, however, and in the majority of joint-working scenarios I felt our value base was aligned. Where conflict of opinion or direct professional challenge occurred, again this could be daunting but largely a valid and valuable position to hold in professional practice. Returning to the concept of experiential knowledge, diversity in the interprofessional model of welfare practice potentially challenges the traditions of formal knowledge and a tension is valued if it creates reflection and new knowledge based on diversity of perspectives.

Work with managers

I have remained in front-line work with service users and carers rather than taking a managerial post. Inevitably there will be some clashes between front-line practice perspectives and managerial reactions to crises and economic expediency. There are ways of maintaining a managerial role in social work that is still directly in touch with practice arenas, and I value this potential in the profession.

Key learning points

- Knowledge approaches promote a critical appraisal of practice and use of self.
- Social workers practise in partnership with service users and carers, colleagues and managers.
- Social workers adhere to a consistent value base reflecting the GSCC and BASW requirements.
- Open channels of communication that readily acknowledge and raise sources of conflict and diverse opinion are important.
- Social work promotes choice and individual responsibility.

REFLECTION ACTIVITIES

1. How might your own belief system conflict with your work as a people professional?
2. Diggins (2004) highlights key messages from service users and carers about communication skills in social work. Social workers who are good at communication:

   - are courteous;
   - turn up on time;
   - speak directly to service users, not carers or personal assistants;
   - don't use jargon;
   - 'open their ears' and 'think before they talk';
   - listen and 'really hear' and accept what carers are saying;
   - explain what is happening and why;
   - do what they say they are going to do and don't over-promise;
   - say honestly when they can't help;
   - are patient and make enough time to communicate with disabled service users.

   How appropriate do you think this list would be as a charter for all people professionals?

FURTHER READING

Dominelli, L. (2002) 'Anti-oppressive practice in context', in Adams, R., Dominelli, L. and Payne, M. (Eds) *Social Work: Themes, Issues and Critical Debates* (2nd Ed.). London: Stationery Office

Howe, D. (2008) *The Emotionally Intelligent Social Worker*. Basingstoke: Palgrave Macmillan

Miller, L. (2006) *Counselling Skills for Social Work*. London: Sage

Seden, J. (2005) *Counselling Skills in Social Work Practice* (2nd Ed.). Maidenhead: Open University Press

Thompson, N. (2005) *Understanding Social Work: Preparing for Practice* (2nd Ed.). Berkshire: Open University Press

Thompson, S. and Thompson, N. (2008) *The Critically Reflective Practitioner*. Basingstoke: Palgrave Macmillan

Chapter 6

Interpersonal Skills in Mental Health Nursing

Dr Debbie Evans

EDITOR'S INTRODUCTION

The World Health Organisation (WHO, 2001) estimates that one in four people in the world will suffer from a mental health problem at some point in their lives. The key role of a mental health nurse is to form therapeutic relationships with mentally ill people and their families. In common with many people professionals, one of the key skills of a mental health nurse is the power of their own personality, together with effective communication skills and an understanding of the theories associated with mental illness.

In this chapter you will read about the work of a mental health nurse working with those who experience both physical and psychological difficulties as a result of alcohol abuse.

Key themes

- Applying theory to practice.
- Ethics and confidentiality.
- Service user perspective.
- Supervision.

Pre-reading reflection activity

Thorneycroft (2006) suggests that not only is there discrimination against people with a mental illness but that mental health staff are also subjected to a form of 'stigma by association'. How do you think such a stigma would affect the ability of a mental health nurse to develop and sustain effective relationships with service users?

DEBBIE EVANS – MENTAL HEALTH NURSE

Describe the kind of interactions that you might have with people in the course of the normal working day and the theoretical models that underpin your practice

To me the great joy of working in mental health is the opportunity to empower individuals and their supporters to examine the maladaptive choices that underpin their conditions, enabling them to move towards recovery. As there is still no real agreement about what causes mental illness, support exists for a whole range of interpretations, which range from the medical model, where mental illness is a biological process, to **humanistic** interpretations, where mental illness is a failure to self-actualise. Because of this, practitioners have to carefully consider what they believe, which models of mental health and nursing they subscribe to, as this will influence the interactions they have with the client group. My practice draws upon the synthesis of two models, these being Peplau's model of care and person-centred approaches to facilitating change.

Peplau (1992) stated that nursing is a significant interpersonal process that aims to promote a patient's health in the direction of creative, constructive, productive, community living. The crux of nursing is that it promotes this growth within a nurse–client relationship. The relationship develops through overlapping phases until resolution, when the client will be independent and well again. Peplau (1992) stated that these phases are orientation, identification, exploration and resolution (see Figure 1).

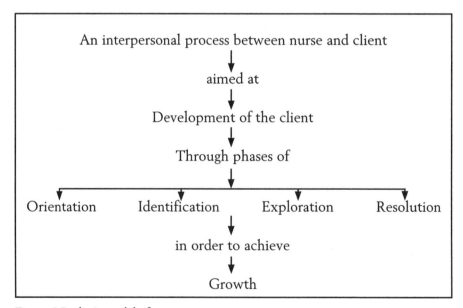

Figure 1 Peplau's model of care

Peplau (1992) stated that orientation is the phase where the client and the nurse learn the nature of the difficulty that the client is experiencing and they work towards a mutual trust. It is at this stage of the interpersonal relationship that information is collected in order that the problems can be identified. The identification phase is reached when the client recognises that a relationship is being formed and they plan together the appropriate interventions. Peplau believed that nurses have expert knowledge and that the responsibility lies with the nurse to formulate the plans and goals. The nurse uses their expert knowledge to help the client gain a better understanding and insight into their particular difficulty. The exploration phase occurs when the client recognises and responds to the services that are offered by the nurse. The interpersonal process is fully utilised and the client moves into action to achieve the mutually recognised goals. The resolution phase occurs when the tension is resolved and the client no longer requires nursing intervention. The client has grown and has achieved independence.

Peplau believed that in order to facilitate the process of orientation to exploration it was necessary to recognise different roles and skills. These roles can be specific to particular parts of the process, such as that of stranger, or used throughout, such as that of teacher.

The role of stranger relates to the beginning of the interpersonal process and recognises that the nurse and the client are strangers to each other. The client will be treated with respect and courtesy. Peplau (1992) reminds us that we should treat the client as emotionally able, unless there is evidence to indicate otherwise. When in the role of resource person the nurse provides specific answers to questions. As a teacher the nurse has two choices: to give information, which Peplau calls instructional, or to be experimental, where the nurse uses the client's experience as a basis from which learning is developed. As a leader the nurse helps the client meet the tasks in hand through a relationship of co-operation and active participation. The nurse can also act as a surrogate. The nurse's attitudes and behaviour trigger responses that reflect reactivated feelings from a prior relationship – referred to as transference. When this occurs the nurse's role is to assist the client to identify these feelings and to offload and ventilate them in a healthy fashion. It would be necessary to engage in a counselling relationship, the purpose of which would be to enable the client to remember and understand fully what is happening in the present situation so that the experience can be integrated into rather than dissociated from the experiences of life.

The model suggests that you are most likely to be in the stranger role at the beginning of the relationship. It also suggests that the client will move from infant through to adult as they move through the phases and resolve their problem. You are most likely to be the resource person and counsellor as you move into identification and exploration. When the client achieves independence in the resolution stage, then both you and the client will be in an adult relationship.

Having a model of care is very helpful, as it provides a theoretical base for your care delivery. However, it is meaningless unless you utilise the correct skills and demonstrate the correct attitudes to allow the client to engage in the process of change.

What are the key skills that you use in your work with people?

Rogers (1959) suggests that there are core conditions, which I refer to as attitudes, that need to be in place in order for a client to engage in that process of actualisation. These attitudes are empathy, congruence and a non-judgemental approach. He would argue that, to some extent, it is not what you do, it's the way that you do it. With regard to the skills that we need to facilitate change, some are constant throughout such as Egan's (1998) SOLER micro skills. These are skills that assist the practitioner to attend to the client and are vital throughout every interaction we have. SOLER is an acronym that stands for:

S – face the client and sit Squarely. (You may need to adjust this based on cultural norms. For example, in Asian cultures a woman sitting directly opposite to a man is seen as aggressive.)
O – adopt an Open posture as this communicates openness and availability to the client.
L – Lean towards the other as this non-verbally shows that you are interested in what the person has to say.
E – maintain good Eye contact, but do not stare. Personally I found that I developed this skill by imagining a grid on the person's face and then slowly scanning that. It became instinctive after a short period of time.
R – be Relaxed, do not fidget or be distracting.

By becoming proficient in these skills you develop many of the non-verbal skills needed for attending.

Dickinson *et al.* (1989) break down the skills required into phases and refer to them as responding skills, initiating skills and interaction strategies. Responding skills include non-verbal communication, reinforcement, reflecting, listening and self-disclosure. Initiating skills include questioning, explaining and opening and closing. Interactional strategies include influencing, counselling and interviewing. Interaction strategies draw upon the skills within the responding and initiating skills categories.

Responding skills

Reinforcement

Reinforcement is where we encourage the client's involvement and demonstrate interest both verbally and non-verbally in what is being said and done. We can respond non-verbally, for example by utilising SOLER, and verbally by compliments, acknowledgements, and supportive and evaluative comments.

Reassurance

We also provide reassurance, conveying friendliness and warmth, while selectively controlling the topic of conversation when reinforcing particular themes.

Reflection

Reflection is when we decide to focus specifically on themes in the communication that can be either factual or emotional. We do this by utilising the skill of paraphrasing, allowing us to respond to the client, utilising their own words, to provide feedback for them.

Listening

Listening is a critical skill which can be defined as the assimilation of both verbal and non-verbal messages. Listening is an active skill and you need to do it with both your eyes and your ears.

Self-disclosure

The skill of self-disclosure enhances the therapeutic relationship as it conveys genuineness and strengthens interpersonal attraction and social influence. Self-disclosure is used to open conversations, encourage reciprocation, provide reassurance, share common experiences and facilitate self-expression.

When we examine these skills we can see that they fall into the responsive category as they are usually employed in reaction to behaviour.

Initiating skills

The initiating skills in contrast are employed when the practitioner initiates the interaction or has a leading role in it.

Questioning

Questioning is about eliciting accurate information and, at its simplest, is a request for information. Questions are used to gain precise information, to open interactions, to focus a person's attention on a particular area, to assess understanding, to maintain control, to encourage participation, to demonstrate interest and to facilitate discussion. To achieve these aims a range of questions can be used, which include open, closed, leading and probing.

Explaining

Another initiating skill is explaining, which is to give understanding to another. The aim of explaining is to provide information, simplify complexities, correct misinformation, give advice, aid compliance, offer reassurance, justify actions and ensure understanding.

Opening and closing interactions

Opening and closing the interaction is important as people tend to remember what happened first and last in a sequence of events. In the opening phase attention should be paid to meeting, greeting and seating. It is important that at the beginning you set the scene for your client, letting them know what you are going to do, give reasons for what you are doing, answer any questions the client has, explain what is expected of them and gain their cooperation.

In the closing phase you need to ensure that you facilitate a smooth, effective closure. To do this you need to learn to utilise closure indicators and markers such as breaking eye contact. It is very useful to summarise the therapeutic conversation that has taken place as this allows both review and closure. Making future links is another way that you can instigate closure and you are bringing the client into the future.

Interaction strategies

The final category is interaction strategies, which include counselling, interviewing and influencing strategies.

Counselling

Counselling is a therapeutic process that Hopson (1981) describes as:

> Helping someone to explore a problem, clarify conflicting issues and discover alternative ways of dealing with it, so that they can decide what to do about it, that is helping people to help themselves. (p. 267)

Hopson goes on to identify that the main function of counselling is to enter into a relationship where the client feels accepted and understood, to achieve an increased understanding of the situation, to discuss alternative courses of actions, to make decisions about what to do, to draw up plans and do with support, do what is required. We can see that being able to facilitate this process draws upon many of the skills identified in the initiating and responding categories.

Influencing

Influencing is required when a client seems resistant to make the changes required and Dickinson *et al.* (1989) identify a range of influencing tactics. These include the use of power, which can be broken down into expert, informational, legitimate, referent, reward and coercive. There are obviously ethical issues associated with the use of power, which are discussed later in this chapter when I introduce you to David Seedhouse's ethical grid.

Interviewing

The third strategy is interviewing, which ranges from non-structured through to highly structured standardised interviews that would include an assessment. There are five stages whichever type of interviewing you are considering. These are: the pre-interview stage, which is where you ensure you are prepared both practically and psychologically; the opening phase, where you meet, greet and seat your client; the information collection stage, where you utilise skills such as questioning, explaining and paraphrasing; and the closing phase, where you draw the interview to an end, drawing on the skills of summarising.

Working as a nurse who specialises in working with individuals who abuse alcohol, either because of physical or psychological addiction, there is not what you could call a standard day. Often you are working with people who still need to deny the influence alcohol has over their life, alongside those who have made significant changes and have left alcohol behind as a crutch. I have chosen to share Keri's story with you, to show how she progressed through various stages of change until she was able to live without alcohol.

Case study

Keri had been drinking since she was 14 years old. Her drinking became heavier three years later and her GP advised her that she had non-A non-B hepatitis. He advised Keri to abstain from alcohol for six months. Keri was actually able to do this but, when she did stop drinking, she experienced withdrawals (she did not recognise them as such). She started drinking again and her previous drinking pattern took only three days to reinstate, this being approximately 14 pints or 28 units per day. She again began to feel 'ill' and the GP on this occasion homed in on the palpitations and shakes Keri described and highlighted anxiety as the problem. The GP advised Keri that she should not drink to cope with her anxiety and referred her onto a psychologist for anxiety management work. Keri decided she would cut down but the more she tried the more she craved for a drink and really her drinking only ceased for up to 48 hours at any one time. Then her 'anxiety' got too much for her and she returned to alcohol. She knew that alcohol made the horrible physical sensations go away. When she visited the psychologist, Keri was asked in more depth about the timing of her 'panic attacks'. The psychologist did a comprehensive drinking history and explained to Keri that he thought her anxiety was as a direct result of her alcohol consumption and that he was going to refer her to the specialist services. However, Keri was not willing to accept that she had an alcohol problem and she did not keep the appointment with the alcohol services.

One common problem is that many people who have alcohol problems do not keep appointments with the service on offer to them. As a result of this fact the team undertakes to visit everyone who has not kept their outpatient appointment and it was as a result of this initiative that I met Keri.

Keri's assessment took a long time because she was very unsure about having contact with me and she would often not keep appointments.

However, over time it became clear that she drank sufficient alcohol to be considered alcohol dependent, though she herself was unwilling to accept this. She clung onto the fact that she had periods of abstinence so could not be a problem drinker!

Keri put anxiety forward as her primary problem and I agreed that it was important to work towards reducing the amount of anxiety she experienced, but without losing sight of the fact that her alcohol intake may be contributing to this problem. I think the fact that she had consciously stopped taking 'drugs', because she did not want to become addicted, was one of the main reasons she continued to deny her dependence on alcohol so strongly. This is a fact that is voiced very often and one that I personally find very sad. Using Peplau's phases we can see a process that ultimately led to Keri's abstinence from alcohol.

I visited Keri as she was not attending outpatient appointments. It was obvious from her referral letter that she was not willing to accept that alcohol was a problem. Anxiety also seemed to be a problem. A letter was sent explaining that I would visit.

During the first visit Keri was asking questions as to why I was calling. She was reluctant and hesitant to accept assistance. She was adamant that she did not need help, as she had managed to be dry on her own. She reiterated that anxiety was her problem and that, as nobody really cared anyway, I should go away. My responsibilities while in the role of stranger and resource person were to:

- give the parameters of the meeting;
- explain roles and gather data;
- help Keri identify problems;
- work to reduce anxiety and tension;
- focus Keri's energies; and
- clarify preconceptions and expectations of the nurse.

I did this by:

- explaining why I had called, referring back to the referral letter;
- explaining who I was;
- asking why Keri had felt unable to keep her outpatient appointment;

▶

- asking Keri to state what she believed her problems were and what she would like as assistance;
- explaining what was on offer, i.e. clarification of her problems;
- providing education regarding alcohol and its effects;
- examining her anxiety – classifying whether she was suffering withdrawals or not;
- explaining that I was not there to shout at her;
- explaining that I was there to help her with whatever she perceived to be a problem at that time. i.e. starting with the anxiety, even though alcohol was the problem;
- asking her if there was anything she wanted to know about me, e.g. did I drink, how long had I been doing the job, or had I worked with other people before.

To achieve this, the skills and values that I needed to utilise were:

- SOLER;
- core conditions;
- initiating skills;
- responding skills.

Keri moved from orientation into the phase of identification as she began to accept that alcohol might have a part to play in her condition. My role changed as I became a teacher, resource person and leader.

Keri agreed to further visits. However, she tested me out by not keeping some of them as she wanted to see if I would yell at her or if I was bothered enough to keep coming. She became willing to consider that there may be many factors contributing to her anxiety and she recognised the need to clarify the situation. She became more willing to explain and explore her drinking history and patterns. As time progressed she began to understand why I was calling and to utilise the sessions and was able to acknowledge that she did not know anything about alcohol and detoxification. Crucially she began to view me as an individual rather than an authority figure. She also attempted changes and stopped drinking alcohol for a period of time.

My responsibilities as teacher, resource person and leader were to:

- maintain a separate identity;
- help Keri to focus on issues – therapeutically confront defence mechanisms, e.g. denial, rationalisation;
- acknowledge Keri's need to 'check you out';
- demonstrate unconditional acceptance of Keri;
- help Keri to explore, ventilate and offload feelings;
- help Keri to identify needs;
- provide information on alcohol and anxiety;
- provide information that helped Keri 'identify' triggers;
- provide information about alternative behaviours;
- work on Keri's use of language (taking responsibility).

I did this by:

- not reacting negatively when Keri did not keep appointments;
- taking a full drinking history and doing a full assessment – creating a road map;
- giving basic alcohol and anxiety facts;
- encouraging use of a drink diary to establish patterns and triggers;
- offering alternatives to triggers;
- using reflection and paraphrasing to help Keri clarify her needs;
- using a non-judgemental approach – not placing a value on Keri's feelings;
- reframing Keri's 'can't' and 'you' to 'won't' and 'I'.

To achieve this, the skills and values I needed to utilise were:

- SOLER;
- core conditions;
- initiating skills;
- responding skills;
- interactional strategies.

Keri moved into exploration as she actively began to change her drinking behaviours and recognised that alcohol was indeed the primary concern. My role changed again as I became the leader and surrogate. Keri began to be more open and flexible, kept all appointments and did her homework. She began to appreciate that it is possible to 'enjoy' life without alcohol and acknowledged the need for abstinence and more intensive detoxification and treatment. My responsibilities, while in the leader and surrogate roles, were to:

▶

- continue to meet Keri's needs as they emerged;
- understand and clarify shifts in behaviour;
- initiate long-term treatment goals;
- identify and reinforce positive factors;
- facilitate forward movement in personality – deal with denial, etc.;
- deal with therapeutic impasses and transference issues.

I did this by:

- continuing to recap and reinforce alcohol facts;
- encouraging family members and friends not to collude with drinking behaviour;
- offering positives;
- supporting new understanding as to why she had not been able to stop on her own;
- reinforcing the realities and dangers of stopping without support;
- reinforcing what facilities are open to her;
- dealing with 'blocks' as they emerge;
- acknowledging the need to 'regress' but not reacting, using this as a positive learning experience.

To achieve this, the values and skills I needed to utilise were:

- SOLER;
- core conditions;
- initiating skills;
- responding skills;
- interactional strategies.

This process took place over a six-month period. She spent approximately two months in the orientation stage, not believing anyone cared about what happened to her and consequently not trusting me. Within the orientation phase Keri was very hesitant and scared. She saw me as a figure from the establishment and as a threat to her drinking. In this phase the roles I undertook were stranger and resource person. Within the identification stage Keri began to interact, testing me out and then beginning to place some value on what I had to offer. She began to use the information and link anxiety with withdrawals. We were able to establish the need for abstinence and begin to provide information about detoxification. At this stage the main issue was her fear of the detoxification process. I arranged for her to meet other clients who had undergone detoxification. In this phase the roles I undertook were resource person, teacher and leader.

In the exploration phase she began to make moves to become abstinent and agreed to make contact with the outpatients department and undergo detoxification. In this phase the role I undertook was that of leadership. Keri went through a traumatic detoxification that was at its height for about two days. She then craved for at least two months.

When she moved onto the day unit, I was very much in the surrogate role while other members of staff were strangers to her. I therefore remained her key worker during her participation in the unit programme. She had explained that she had felt abandoned when she commenced the programme and that this was a familiar feeling. Keri successfully underwent the programme offered on the Problem Drinking Unit and remains abstinent.

What is the legislative framework that underpins your practice and what are the ethical issues that impact on your practice?

Work of this type is hugely rewarding. However, it is not without its demands. The first set of demands I would like to focus upon are the legislative and ethical frameworks which underpin my practice, and the ways in which they impact on practice.

As a nurse my practice is regulated by the Nursing and Midwifery Council (NMC), which sets out standards for conduct, performance and ethics. The standards can be found in the document called *Protecting the Public through Professional Standards* (2004b). The code covers seven areas and states that we must:

- respect the patient or client as an individual;
- obtain consent before giving any treatment or care;
- protect confidential information;
- co-operate with others in the team;
- maintain professional knowledge and competence;

- be trustworthy; and
- act to identify and minimise risk to patients and clients.

None of these is particularly problematic, perhaps with the exception of 'protect confidential information', which often creates debate within mental health. When a client arrived drunk at the Problem Drinking Unit, we would ask them to leave. If they had come by car we would ask them to give us their car keys. This was always a contentious issue. Some staff would insist on maintaining confidentiality, letting the client leave and drive, risking an accident, while others would want to call the police to have them stopped from driving. Clearly this is not a straightforward issue and, until I discovered the 'ethical grid', I could never decide what to do.

The ethical grid

The ethical grid (Seedhouse, 1988) is a tool that allows you to consider a range of factors and aids the choice of actions that will produce the highest degree of morality (see Figure 2). Seedhouse states:

> The ethical grid is not a tool, in the way that a conveyor belt is a tool; rather it is like a spade that the gardener will use to cultivate his land. The grid does not deliver the correct answer in the way that conveyor belts can be used to deliver neat packages. Like a good gardener the proficient user of the ethical grid will understand his need to keep the tool as clean and as sharp as possible, and he will also know the best way in which to use the tool in order to get the best out of the situation, and in order that the material on which he is working will be treated in the best way possible. (p.127)

As you can see in Figure 2, the grid is made up of four layers and each layer includes a series of boxes. The boxes are independent and detachable. The four layers represent four different elements that make up ethical deliberation. The way to use the grid is to start with the innermost layer, where the boxes identify the basis of health care that is the core of what practitioners engage in, and then move out towards the outermost layer, asking yourself questions as you go, guided by the boxes in each layer, in order to come to a conclusion about the care you wish to deliver. We will consider below each layer separately.

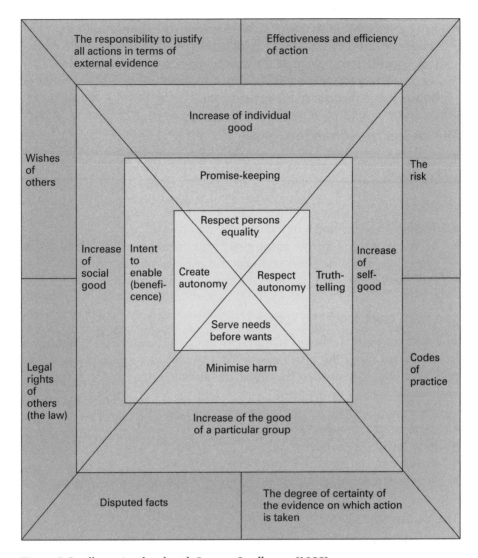

Figure 2 Seedhouse's ethical grid. Source: Seedhouse (1988).

The innermost layer

The four boxes in the innermost layer are:

- *Create autonomy* – a reminder that all clients are individuals who have the capacity to choose freely for themselves.
- *Respect autonomy* – respect an individual's choice, however contentious and difficult. The core of this ideal is that I must ensure that their choices are based upon accurate information.
- *Respect persons equally* – being able to values one's life and having potential for future choices are qualities shared equally by all persons.

- *Serve needs before wants* – is based upon the assumption that the services must provide for the basic needs of all those it seeks to serve. It is important to recognise the difference between needs and wants – we 'need' oxygen to sustain life and although I 'want' a beautiful large house, it is unnecessary for my survival.

The second layer from the centre

The next layer of the grid and the boxes within it are based upon duties and motive:

- *Beneficence* – a duty to do good and to prevent harm.
- *Truth-telling* – telling a lie takes away a person's liberty.
- *Minimise harm* – aim to minimise harm, rather than do no harm, as some actions in the short term can be considered harmful.
- *Promise-keeping* – this demonstrates respect for people.

The third layer from the centre

The next layer and the boxes within it focus upon consequences. Whatever issue you are using the grid for, it is vital to consider consequences. The grid asks you to consider the most beneficial outcome for a range of individuals broken down into:

- increase of individual good;
- increase of self-good;
- increase of the good of a particular group; and
- increase of social good.

The outermost layer

The final layer focuses upon external considerations. These include:

- the responsibility to justify all actions in terms of the evidence, encouraging the practitioner to ensure that care is evidence based;
- effectiveness and efficiency of action, again utilising evidence to show that what you propose is effective;
- the risk;
- codes of practice such as the Nursing and Midwifery Code of Professional Conduct, including requirements such as to protect confidential information –
  see **www.nmc-uk.org/aArticle.aspx?ArticleID=3056**
- the degree of certainty of the evidence on which action is taken – which reminds you to check that you do fully appreciate the situation;
- disputed facts – often family members will provide you with

conflicting information so, as a practitioner, you need to be able to draw upon all the information to exclude inaccurate reporting;

- the law – this may not always coincide with what you believe is correct; something can be lawful yet immoral and vice versa;
- the wishes of others.

So, if I return to our problem drinker who has driven while significantly under the influence of alcohol and refused to give up the keys, the options are:

- to maintain confidentiality, allowing them to leave with their keys;
- to breach confidentiality and alert the police to their condition.

The innermost layer of the grid reminds me that I must respect the autonomy of the client and their decision to drive. However, I must also respect the autonomy of the general public, who may be involved in an accident. My main responsibility is to maintain the client's safety.

I move on to the next layer and am reminded that I need to minimise harm and that we need to be beneficent – do good to prevent harm. The next layer out reminds me that we need to increase the good of the individual and the particular group of road users he would come into contact with. The outermost layer reminds me about our responsibilities under law, the risk, the responsibilities and wishes of others.

The decision of the team was that we would ensure that there were posters up in the Unit, saying that if people did not surrender their car keys when they had been drinking then we would call the police. We wrote it into their contracts and, therefore, when they did this they knew the consequences so it was part of their own decision-making. Although, technically, we were breaching confidentiality, we were acting in a way to protect them and other road users and were being congruent with what we had said we would do.

Working with people can be very demanding. How do you care for yourself and how do you manage the conflicting demands of working with service users, colleagues and managers?

You will have seen from Keri's case study that this is very demanding work. It is emotionally charged work and you can often find yourself dealing with conflicting needs: those of the client, the managers and your colleagues. Working in any service means that there is often a clash between the organisational culture and the needs of the clients. It does seem ironic that people tend to come into nursing because they want to help people, yet we need to be sick before this help can be accessed. Clinical decision making is affected by a whole range of factors, which include organisational factors, desire for status and fear of challenge.

Much is written from the service user and carer perspective about their needs not being respected and many conclude that the focus of the organisation is to maintain its own survival. One of the tools that you can use to ensure that the client's agenda remains in the forefront is the Ten Essential Shared Capabilities for Mental Health Practice (DoH, 2004b). These focus upon:

- working in partnership with the client and any other person who is significant in their life;
- respecting diversity, recognising that we are all different;
- practising ethically;
- challenging inequality;
- promoting recovery;
- identifing people's needs and strengths;
- providing service user-centred care;
- making a difference;
- promoting safe and positive risk taking and
- ensuring your own personal development and learning.

Using a model of care can help you explain to others that care strategies are legitimate. Peplau's model allows you to legitimatise the client's dependency on the nurse. It has always been my belief that for a person to move forwards they are going to experience a degree of dependency on the nurse. By explaining the different types of 'closeness', it has clarified for me what is enabling and what is inhibiting in the care process. There is a movement within psychiatry that sees dependency as negative and proposes that the key worker should be changed. I now know that dependency is legitimate and it is how we respond as nurses that either complicates or clarifies the situation for the client. To change Keri's key worker when she moved into the Problem Drinking Unit would have reinforced her beliefs about people misusing her trust.

How do you ensure that your practice responds to current research?

Clinical supervision is one way of ensuring that I maintain my integrity as a practitioner. The NMC (2006a) identified that the NHS Management Executive defined clinical supervision as:

A formal process of professional support and learning that enables individual practitioners to develop knowledge and competence, assume responsibility for their own practice and enhance consumer protection and safety in complex situations. (p. 1)

The Mental Health Nursing Association (1995) takes this further to describe the relationship and defines clinical supervision as a

. . . dynamic, interpersonally focused experience which promotes the development of therapeutic proficiency. One of the primary reasons for all supervision is to ensure that the quality of therapeutic intervention with the client is of a consistently high standard in relation to the client's needs. Consequently, supervision must be acknowledged as a cornerstone of clinical practice. (p.1)

Wolsey and Leach (1997) suggest that the process of clinical supervision is an exploration of the difficulty you are encountering, which leads to a new understanding, perhaps around transference, which allows you to re-engage with the client in a different way. Clinical supervision is therefore useful as it allows you to focus upon issues that affect the client's journey, which may be about the client, you and your knowledge, skill or attitudinal base or the organisation you work in, and to develop research options, strategies and interventions.

My experience of clinical supervision is that it is particularly helpful when dealing with **transference** and **counter-transference** and developing emotional intelligence. Transference is the unconscious transfer to others of feelings and attitudes that were originally associated with important figures (parents, siblings, etc.) in one's early life. This manifests itself when you experience what seems, for example, to be inappropriate levels of anger from the client. When you delve into their responses, you discover the behaviour was fuelled by a mannerism you have that reminded them of a much feared aunt. We as practitioners can also do this to our clients; I remember a particularly difficult therapeutic relationship that was confusing to me because he reminded me of my father. This is called **counter-transference**. Clinical supervision is useful when this arises as it allows you to consider your behaviour within the nurse patient relationship.

Another factor that can affect the therapeutic relationship is your level of emotional intelligence. Goleman (1996) states that there is an ABC of emotional intelligence, which has as its main components self-awareness, personal decision-making, managing feelings, empathy, communication, self-disclosure, insight, self-acceptance, personal responsibility, assertiveness, group skills and conflict resolution.

As nurses we are human beings as well, with all our personal-intra personal difficulties. Rogers (1970) wrote:

> As a person, the nurse is continually interacting with her personal (intra personal) environment, as a professional she is continually interacting with the professional environment. Because the human develops the personal self first, that personally organised set of behaviours forms the basis of the self brought into the profession. The personal self is highly influential on the emerging professional self. Understanding self and working to view self more positively inevitably leads to a more productive professional self concept. Negative self concepts are barriers to the effective independent functioning vital to the successful performance of professional roles. (p. 41)

How are your continuing professional development needs fulfilled?

So, you can see that during clinical supervision you are very likely to recognise that you have deficits in your theoretical knowledge or skills base as well as your own intra-personal functioning. Some practitioners would see this as a failure. However, in reality, we are human and we cannot know everything. What is important is that we recognise the need to continue learning, about our professional knowledge, ourselves and the world we live in and that we act on those needs by engaging in activities such as educational courses, conferences, reading, support groups, work in the clinical arena and, when necessary, personal counselling. To ensure that I do not lose touch with practice I hold an honorary contract with the local NHS Trust and return to practice for approximately two weeks per year.

Key learning points

- Mental health nursing is a rewarding career.
- Effective interactions depend upon your ability to work therapeutically with people.
- A model of care can provide a framework for therapeutic relationship building.
- Change is facilitated through a process that takes time to proceed.
- Knowledge is not enough: you need to develop a repertoire of skills and demonstrate facilitative attitudes.
- Care is delivered within a legislative and ethical framework.
- Clinical supervision is a useful support strategy; it allows you to explore difficulties you are having with a client and to further develop your knowledge, skills and attitudes as necessary.
- This is emotionally demanding work and you must ensure that your psychological needs are met as part of the process.

REFLECTIVE ACTIVITIES

1. What would you do if you knew that a service user was going to drive home when it is evident to you that they have had too much to drink?
2. Think about a situation where you have struggled to know what the right thing to do was. Try to work it through using Seedhouse's ethical grid.
3. Goleman (1996) said that a person with high emotional intelligence was more capable of understanding the feelings of others. Do you think this is true? You can take a 'quiz' online to identify your emotional intelligence. Considering the questions that it contains will enable you to begin the process of exploring your own reactions to emotional issues. Go to **www.queendom.com/tests/access_page/ index.htm?idRegTest=11**.

RECOMMENDED READING

Department of Health (2004) *The Ten Essential Shared Capabilities – A Framework for the Whole of the Mental Health Workforce.* London: Department of Health

Dickinson, D.A., Hargie, O. and Morrow, N.C. (1989) *Communication Skills Training for Health Care Professionals.* London: Chapman & Hall

Egan, G. (1990) *The Skilled Helper. A Systematic Approach to Effective Helping* (4th Ed.). Belmont, CA: Brooks/Cole

Chapter 7

Interpersonal Skills in Nursing

Lisa Collicott

EDITOR'S INTRODUCTION

In this chapter you will learn about the work of a senior staff nurse in the Emergency Response and Critical Care Outreach Team in a large central London teaching hospital. In common with other practitioners represented in this text Lisa deals with life and death situations. She may need to tell someone that their loved one has died as well as cope with her own emotions at being with someone at the end of their life. Those with whom she works will be at their most vulnerable.

Advances in medicine mean that patients spend much less time in hospital than ever before, making it even more challenging to build and sustain positive relationships.

Key themes

- Diversity.
- Continuing professional development.
- Supervision.
- Evidence-based practice.

Pre-reading reflection activity

Think about a time when you have felt unwell and needed the help of a health professional. What were their interpersonal skills like?

LISA COLLICOTT – SENIOR STAFF NURSE

Describe the kind of interactions that you might have with people in the course of a normal working day

My work involves daily caring for patients on both the Intensive Care Unit (ICU) and the wards, working with a large multidisciplinary team (MDT) and managing an ever-changing caseload of patients. As an Expanded Role Nurse who is on-call and on the cardiac arrest teams, I cover all departments and areas of the hospital, so I must be able to communicate and work effectively with all levels of staff including medical, nursing and the MDT, often during stressful or emergency situations.

In the course of a normal day I have countless interactions with a variety of people, all requiring different communication skills to acquire and provide information and assess situations. These include the following.

Communicating with colleagues

Handing over information from one shift to the next is imperative to the safety and continuity of care provided to patients. If vital information is not handed over adequately the next nurse will not know essential details about the patient and their care. The most important elements of communicating effectively with colleagues in my role are:

- **Clarity** – being concise allows the other person to identify which details are most important. This is difficult to do when giving a lot of information in a small amount of time and the other person may not know the patient you are referring to. Never assume that a colleague or patient knows what you are referring to or what you are asking them. Being clear with questions and requests will help to avoid confusion or misunderstanding.
- **Prioritising** – providing the most important information first emphasises to others that the information is significant. Effective prioritisation of information is a skill that comes with experience.

Communicating with patients

To effectively communicate with patients I find it helpful to remember the following:

- Introductions help to reduce patients' anxiety of strangers.
- Although acronyms are commonplace throughout medicine and nursing, it can frighten patients and make them think we are trying to hide something from them. Use clear language when speaking to and

in front of patients and relatives to allow patients to feel part of the decision-making process. Imagine the effect on a patient of hearing a doctor say 'Nurse, could you take an FBC to check for Hb, then pass an NGT, take a BM and ECG, make sure the pt is NBM, check their GCS and prepare the pt for their CT, MRI and CXR?'

- Asking clear questions secures the information required more easily. Open questions such as: 'Hi Mr Johnston, how are you?' invites answers such as 'Fine, thanks, how are you?', 'OK', 'I slept quite well thanks', 'Oh, you know!' Closed questions like 'Do you have any pain this morning, Mr Johnston?' or 'Do you need any more painkillers?' focus the patient on a 'yes' or 'no' answer that provides the best possible information in the shortest time.

Barriers to communication

Patients are often in pain, scared, in a new environment and may never have been in hospital before. Sensitivity, caring and empathy help to build relationships and facilitate good communication but, even so, there are barriers to positive communication including:

- pain;
- hunger;
- lack of understanding.

All of these can cause anger and defensiveness and inhibit effective communication. The effects can be minimised by:

- keeping patients informed of changes to their care;
- answering their questions to the best of your ability;
- explaining what you are going to do before you do it;
- allowing time for questions before you start;
- obtaining verbal consent for procedures.

In the ICU the environment can be distressing to patient and relative alike: 'All critically ill patients are stressed to a greater or lesser degree during their time in intensive care. There is a limit to the stress that each person can tolerate' (Adam and Osborne, 2005). ICU nurses work to reduce patient stress by explaining procedures in an understandable way before undertaking them, supporting the patient emotionally and trying to reduce the amount of noise the patient is exposed to (although ICU is well known to be a noisy environment). Recently, on our unit, we introduced sleep masks and ear plugs to try to improve the quality of the patients' sleep, therefore hopefully allowing them the best opportunity during the day to exercise, meet nutritional needs and recover.

Language can be a significant factor when communicating with patients. If people cannot understand or make themselves understood it is difficult to provide or obtain information adequately. Often sign language or symbolising what you are trying to get across will work in the short term but, for important information, using an interpreter is essential, with translator phone lines being a very valuable service. Resist the temptation to use family members to interpret information as you cannot be certain how they are choosing to word the information to their relative and it could cause misunderstandings. Avoid ambiguity and be honest with patients and relatives; if they ask a question, tell them the answer or find someone who can. If the patient asks a serious or difficult question about their condition or treatment, speak to the senior nurse or ask the doctor to speak to them. It is important to make sure that the patient gets the information or they may become understandably anxious and angry.

Cultural or ethnic differences can be perceived as barriers but, by involving myself and asking questions, I can usually bridge the cultural divide and learn about other people and their cultures.

What are the key skills that you use in your work with people?

A range of interpersonal skills are integral to my practice as a nurse:

- Non-verbal communication is a key tool – it can be a case of what you don't say!
- Eye contact is a powerful tool and can demonstrate togetherness, honesty and concern.
- Body language is particularly important when giving serious information. I sit next to the patient on a chair, at their height, close to them but without touching, and maintaining eye contact.
- Touch must be used appropriately. It can be a powerful tool when comforting and reassuring. By putting my hand on the patient's arm I can often provide a sense of security that words cannot, but only use touch when you are sure it is appropriate or if the patient reaches for your hand.
- Patience is essential. If a patient is deaf or hard of hearing they will need written information. It may be necessary to explain information more than once until it is understood. Having family members with you while you explain what medications are or how and when to take them is helpful as they can reiterate the point when you have gone or when they are at home. There may also be picture boards available, where the patient can point at a symbol to indicate what they need.

- The ability to prioritise is an essential skill in nursing; it allows you to work more effectively while doing the most important jobs first. However, it can be challenging to prioritise when you don't understand which jobs are the most important. When you are a student nurse, or a newly qualified staff nurse, every job seems important and you will do one job at a time often in the order that it is given to you. As a more experienced nurse you will gain an overview of your patients, other nurses' patients, the relatives, your colleagues and the running of the ward as a whole.

- Listening to patients is not just about hearing what your patient is saying, but about giving your patient time to express worries or concerns that they may have. Listening involves being aware of what patients don't say, through non-verbal communication. Facial expressions, hand gestures and posture can often express emotions that the patient may have difficulty verbalising. Maximise your listening skills by paraphrasing the patient's thoughts and expressing understanding of their feelings (Bush, 2001).

- Building empathy enables me to recognise and try to understand something that is affecting the patient. It is about imagining yourself the other person's shoes (Egan, 1998).

- Leadership: in leading by example and always striving for excellence of care I can act as a role model for my peers, junior nurses and other health care professionals that I come into contact with. As workloads increase there is a risk that standards will suffer, but it is essential that patients receive good quality care and that any changes/ deterioration in their condition are identified and a senior nurse or doctor notified.

- Support: be aware of your colleagues and when they may need help, support or merely a break. By being observant assistance can be offered when it is needed, hopefully stopping a stressful situation worsening or avoiding it altogether. Be aware of your patients' relatives; they regularly visit for long periods at a time, often without adequate sleep, nutrition or hydration. Add to that a stressful and upsetting situation of a loved one being in hospital ill and the relative is at risk of becoming unwell themselves. Encouraging your patients' relatives to take regular breaks and meals and enough fluid to drink will all help to create a healthy environment for your patient to recover in.

- Advocacy: 'Nurses have a responsibility to maintain a safe environment for care, maintain patient confidentiality and privacy' (Perrin Ouimet and McGhee, 2001). As a patient's nurse, you are expected to protect the patient when vulnerable, ensure their safety, facilitate them getting the information or support that they may need and speaking up for the patient if they are not able to do so for themselves. If a patient hasn't understood information that a doctor has given them or you think they would benefit from information from a specialist, you can work for the patient to facilitate that.

- Be enthusiastic. Inspire people and work to create a positive work environment. This makes an effective setting for recovery and good well-being for the patients. It can also help to reduce nurses' stress, mental exhaustion and ultimately burnout (Begat and Severinsson, 2006).
- Caring is a core concept of nursing. Patients are nursed and provided with unconditional care, in a non-judgemental way.
- Confidentiality is essential as patients often have illnesses or problems that they do not wish their relatives or other patients to know about. This is their right. Patients' information and details should only be available and accessible to individuals who are authorised to have access to them. There is a large multidisciplinary team working in hospitals from physiotherapists to psychiatric liaison officers and as a patient's nurse it is my responsibility to ensure that the teams or individuals that see the patient and their notes should be seeing them. For confidentiality reasons, it is not appropriate to nurse patients whom we know personally. A colleague should be discreetly asked to take over their care, maintaining confidentiality at all times.
- Be assertive without being aggressive. Sometimes assistance or help is required with a patient and, if everyone else is very busy and not listening to your concerns, it can be difficult to express what you need clearly to the right people. Getting angry or upset doesn't help (no matter how frustrated you are!). Stay calm and be very clear. For example: 'Mrs Clark has suddenly become very drowsy. I am concerned she may have had another stroke. I am very worried. Her blood pressure is 195/120 and her mouth is drooping on the left' would be more likely to elicit the desired response than:

  > Nurse: 'Mrs Clark isn't herself today, she hardly ate any lunch. She's very sleepy.'
  > Doctor: 'I'm busy clerking patients, can it wait until later?'
  > Nurse: 'Can't you come now? You are always busy when I call you!'
  > Doctor: 'I'll come later, when I'm finished here.'

The more information you can provide to other people in the most concise manner possible will assist in getting your point across and allow them to make an informed decision of how urgently they need to get there. If you are not able to adequately assess if the patient has deteriorated or is seriously unwell, give the information you are concerned about to someone who is experienced to use it. If you know something is wrong and you are not sure what it is, inform the nurse in charge and let them, as more experienced practitioners, assess the seriousness of the situation.

What is the legislative framework that underpins your practice?

The nursing profession places delivery of quality health care as its highest goal. The Nursing and Midwifery Council (NMC) works to safeguard the health and well-being of the public by continually regulating, reviewing and promoting nursing and midwifery standards. As the governing body of nursing in the UK all nurses and midwives are registered with the NMC. The NMC governs registered nurses, midwives and specialist community public health nurses. The NMC recently implemented (1 May 2008) an updated version of the *NMC Code of Standards of Conduct, Performance and Ethics for Nurses and Midwives* (NMC, 2008a). It tells me that I am personally accountable for my practice and that in caring for patients and clients I must:

- treat people as individuals and respect their dignity;
- obtain consent before giving any treatment or care;
- respect people's right to confidentiality;
- co-operate with others in the team;
- listen to the people in my care and respond to their concerns;
- keep clear and accurate records;
- recognise and work within the limits of my competence.

The NMC provides advice and information to nurses and midwives on professional standards and considers allegations of misconduct, lack of competence or unfitness to practise. The practising nurse is also accountable in criminal law and civil law.

The development of traditional nurse roles, together with the reduction of doctors' hours (Dowling *et al.*, 1995), has led to nurses having extended roles from critical care outreach to nurse practitioners now being commonplace in our hospitals. With these increasing roles and responsibilities comes increasing accountability. Roles must be clearly defined to allow professionals to work safely within their scope of practice. Nurses who practise outside of those limits are at risk of not being covered by their Trust for vicarious liability (McHale and Tingle, 2007) in case of complaint or legal action.

What theoretical models underpin your practice?

'Nursing theories provide the critical thinking structures to direct the clinical decision-making process of professional practice' (George, 2001). There are many published nursing frameworks, all with different focuses, each being used by different specialities. When Peplau first published her book in 1952 it was considered to be radical for the time. She focused on the interpersonal process, encouraging the nurse to explore mutual expectations and goals with patients. The nurse is involved in a process of self-fulfilment but the main focus is interaction. This model has most significance for mental health nursing. (You can read more about Peplau's model in Chapter 6 on mental health nursing.)

Orem's (2001) theory is that nursing is needed when the self-care demands are greater than the self-care abilities, with the nurse providing assistance only when the individual is unable to care for themselves. This model is most usually applied in community and rehabilitation nursing.

The Roper *et al.* (1996) model of nursing care is based upon the patients' Activities of Living (AL) and is prevalent throughout adult nursing in the UK. It identifies 12 ALs which provide the framework for the patient's assessment on admission, allowing the nurses to ensure their patient's care is individualised to them (Holland, 2003). This model is frequently used for general adult nursing. The ALs are undertaken by individuals daily and each person has a certain ability to perform these activities depending on their health or ill health as indicated by the independence/dependence continuum. An initial assessment is made when a person first enters the hospital, with any deficits in their ability to meet their ALs being part of the nursing care plan to be met by nursing care or patient assistance as required. Since health is dynamic and ever changing, assessment must be a continuous, ongoing process. In the case study below you will be able to see how the Roper *et al.* model is applied in practice.

Case study

Mrs Brown was electively admitted to hospital for a knee operation. She had been well at home but, after complaining of knee pain after a recent ski trip, her GP had diagnosed some ligament damage that would require surgery to examine and repair. On initial assessment Mrs Brown was entirely independent in her ALs but, on assessment after the surgery, the nurse found:

Problem: Maintaining a safe environment. Mrs Brown is unable to transfer from bed to chair without assistance as she has a leg brace on and is in pain.

Plan: She will require assistance from one nurse to transfer.

Problem: Personal cleansing and dressing. Mrs Brown is unable to meet her hygiene needs independently, due to pain and her leg brace.

Plan: She will require assistance to meet hygiene needs.

Problem: Mobilising. Mrs Brown has crutches and is not confident using them.

Plan: The physiotherapist will work with Mrs Brown to assist her becoming competent and confident with mobilising with crutches, including using stairs.

Problem: Sleeping. Mrs Brown is concerned how she will sleep with her leg brace on.

Plan: Reassurance is given that the nurses will help her get comfortable and will provide pain relief when required.

As patients' health improves, their independence with their ALs will improve, which is why ongoing assessment is essential so that the needs of the patients are met adequately, but patients are encouraged to meet the needs they are able to be independent with as they improve.

At the core of my practice as a nurse is an appreciation of Maslow's Hierarchy of Needs. Maslow (1970) identified physiological needs that have to be satisfied before other needs can be met. Basic needs such as food, water and oxygen need to be satisfied before other needs become important. Consider trying to study when all you can think of is which sandwich to make for lunch, or how difficult it is to work if you feel cold. Similarly, patients will find it challenging to understand important information or go the rehabilitation gym when they have just missed lunch, didn't sleep well or are in pain.

What are the ethical issues that impact on your practice?

Ethics attempts to answer the question 'what should I do?' (Perrin Ouimet and McGhee, 2001). As a nurse I am involved with many different people each day, so ethical issues are likely to be part of my everyday work. There are a number of key principles.

Confidentiality

As I have discussed earlier, it is essential for nurses to provide patients with the confidence that their conditions and treatment details will only be accessed by those who need to know. Talking to peers about patients' details is not acceptable; imagine sitting on a bus and hearing a nurse behind you discussing her patients' confidential information with her friend.

When a patient tells you something in confidence that might be detrimental to them, such as thoughts of suicide or of harming others, it is essential to tell the nurse in charge or the patient's doctor so that further action can be taken to protect the patient (or others). Initially this may seem to conflict with patient confidentiality, but it is essential to protect the patient from harm (see non-maleficence). It might be easier if a patient asks you if they can tell you something in confidence to say: 'If it is information that I need to tell a doctor for your own health or that of others, then I will have to do so'. This is especially important if you suspect a child or a vulnerable adult to be in danger as a nurse must comply with the Children Acts 1989 and 2004 and the Mental Capacity Act 2005. The nurse in charge will know whom to contact in this circumstance and it is essential it is reported as soon as possible.

Beneficence

Nurses should always act with beneficence, which means to do good, to avoid evil and to act in the interest of others. There is fine balance to be achieved between beneficence and autonomy as it is important not to deny the patient the autonomy of doing things for themselves with the ultimate aim of recovering and going home.

Non-maleficence

Non-maleficence means to do no harm (Hendrick, 2000) and is based on the ancient Hippocratic Oath. Its aim was to remind physicians to consider the possible harm that an intervention might have on a patient. This would cover avoiding inappropriate relationships with patients, working when unable to do so (for example when under the influence of alcohol) or deliberately causing harm to patients.

Autonomy

The NMC (2008a) states that the patient needs to be respected and supported to accept or decline treatment and care and upholds people's rights to be fully involved in decisions about their care. Patients must therefore give 'informed consent' when undertaking surgery or invasive procedures. The patient must be in possession of the facts and risk factors surrounding the operation or procedure, allowing them the autonomy to make an informed choice whether to have it or not. Patient autonomy is the right of patients to make decisions about their medical care without their health care provider trying to influence the decision, but it must be ensured that the patient is aware of the risks of not having the procedure too. The doctor will have a consent form for the patient to sign if they agree to the procedure and it is the nurse's duty as the patient advocate to ensure that the patient understands the information given to them. If the nurse feels that the patient does not understand they should request that the doctor return and sit with them, reiterating information until it is clear and they can make an informed decision.

A further discussion of the ethical framework for nurses can be found in Beauchamp and Childress (2001). Sometimes, as in the case below of Mr Clarke, a patient will tell you something that they have been unable to tell their family.

Case study

Mr Clarke, an 84-year-old man who had previously been well but had a recent history of feeling generally unwell, was admitted to hospital for blood tests and investigations. The day after the tests Mr Clarke asked whether I knew what was wrong with him and whether it might be something serious like cancer. His history suggested that he had been well until this point so I sat next to him and asked him why he thought it might be cancer. I was able to use my interpersonal skills to help Mr Clarke voice his concerns. He told me that he had suspected it for a while now. He had been feeling unwell for longer than he had told his family, had looked his symptoms up on the internet and was sure he had bowel cancer. He hadn't told his family, as he didn't want them to worry. He said he had lived a good life and hadn't been quite the same since his wife died two years ago from a stroke. She was in the hospital for a long time, had had lots of scans and tests and ended up in intensive care surrounded by equipment with lots of drips. Her heart stopped beating and they tried to save her, but she died. He said he wouldn't want to go through any of that, and was happy to go home and slip away in the night in his own home.

Mr Clarke's family had asked the doctors not to tell their father the results as he would be too distressed by them and that they

▶

would break it gently to him, so when the doctors got the test results back they told the family that their father had advanced bowel cancer and they would offer chemotherapy or radiotherapy if Mr Clarke wanted it for symptom control and to extend life for a month or two. The doctors discussed the patient's resuscitation status in case of sudden deterioration and the family told the doctors they would discuss the chemotherapy option and let them know, but they definitely wanted their father to be resuscitated if his heart was to stop.

I knew Mr Clarke's wishes because I had spoken with him at length and understood that he didn't want to have extensive treatment. I felt that in his position I would probably have the treatment, but I understood it wasn't my place to tell him what I thought. I spoke to Mr Clarke and told him I thought his family wanted to speak to him about his illness and that they were finding it difficult. Mr Clarke's family were surprised that Mr Clarke not only expected the diagnosis, but had a clear plan for his end of life, his understanding of his condition was good and he was fully competent to make these decisions. After an emotional discussion, his family agreed to let Mr Clarke go home with community support from district nurses and cancer specialist nurses.

When he left the hospital Mr Clarke thanked me for supporting his decisions without judging him, for listening and for allowing him to plan a dignified death in his own home.

Putting my own feelings aside and working as his advocate I had helped Mr Clarke to have put in place the arrangements that he wanted. He declined the doctors' treatment plan, but was competent to do so, so could legally choose to go home and be with his family at the end of his life.

You can read more about ethical dilemmas at **www.jcn.co.uk/journal.asp? MonthNum=11&YearNum=2005&Type=backissue&ArticleID=865**

Working with people can be very demanding. How do you care for yourself?

There will inevitably be periods of stress in your career. Nursing involves shift work and this will add to the stressors. Identifying stressors (both yours and other people's) is beneficial to reducing stress. It is important to know when you need to take five minutes away from a discussion if you are upset or angry. Try to remove yourself from the situation, clear your head, then return. This is particularly important if you are affected by the situation you are in (be it giving bad news or coping with upset relatives).

I find **reflection** with colleagues incredibly valuable; it enables me to learn about coping mechanisms from the people that I work with. I can identify what they would do in difficult situations and think about whether it will work for me. We all make mistakes but we can learn from them to build experience for the next situation. Experienced nurses will have seen certain situations before and know what it is helpful to do and how to react. Experience is very valuable in nursing and something that will come with time and exposure to different experiences and situations.

If you require further support and are struggling to find it or need more than you have been offered, most Trusts have a staff support system or access to one. Counsellors are usually accessible.

Being ill at work, even if the ward is very busy, is inadvisable. You may spread whatever you have to other staff or patients. By looking after yourself, you will be better prepared to look after others. For any health concerns the occupational health department offers a wide range of work-related health services, such as immunisations and ongoing health surveillance for the well-being of all staff.

Emergencies happen when you least expect it and, for many nurses, the biggest fear is that a patient suddenly loses consciousness, their vital signs deteriorate and they become unresponsive. As part of the cardiac arrest team I attend these emergency situations and, although we are all trained and proficient in what to do in most situations, it is always advisable to spend time with the patient's nurses when the situation has been controlled in order to discuss and debrief what happened. If there has been a prolonged resuscitation attempt after a cardiac arrest where the patient has not survived, a period of debriefing is always advisable. The nurse may have cared for this patient for days or weeks and have a close relationship with them and their family. Reflecting and debriefing on the positive aspects of the situation allows nurses to develop coping mechanisms while being supported. Informing next of kin and family members of their relative's sudden deterioration is often best managed by a senior nurse with the patient's nurse present, particularly if they have met the relatives before and can provide a familiar face for support.

Debriefing is essential after large-scale emergencies such as major incidents. It will be a formal event, often chaired by a senior manager and involving all the different departments. Counselling is available for all who require it after any such incident.

Clinical supervision is a supportive way to facilitate learning from experience, 'positively influencing existence and well being' (Begat and Severinsson, 2006). It is a formal reflective process, aiming to support and encourage professional growth. During our team days at work, we invite an independent professional, not related to our specialty, who listens confidentially to our concerns and talks through any difficult or challenging situation that we have had. The group then discusses them, offers feedback and suggests possible changes for our future practice. This helps to reduce work-related stress and possible burnout by allowing nurses to learn from previous experiences and plan for the next time it happens.

The medical teams have Morbidity & Mortality presentations. These are medical peer reviews of a patient's case to learn from complications and adverse outcomes to allow for reflection and to identify areas for improvement. Their aim is to benefit patient care in the future.

How do you ensure that your practice responds to current research?

As expanded role nurses, we organise and run regular teaching days for ward nurses, concentrating on the anatomy and physiology of body systems and clinical nursing procedures. We explain, in depth, how things should be done and why. Nurses are able to practise practical skills and ask questions in a learning environment. We will then work on the wards, often undertaking impromptu teaching sessions when situations occur with a procedure or piece of equipment that the nurses are unfamiliar with, and providing continuing support.

Conferences are an excellent way to increase knowledge, as experts in the field will discuss new innovations or changes to treatment or care. They enable delegates from different areas or countries to discuss the innovations and plan how to implement them in their areas of care.

'Journal club' is a monthly meeting of the senior staff, both nursing and medical, where one staff member has identified and presents a research article or topic, which is then discussed in depth. We consider how it applies to our patient base and identify any improvements that we might make to patient care. The ICU has such a wide range of patients, conditions and treatments and, with research being done all over the world all of the time, it is important to keep up to date with large reputable studies and the results or conclusions they have had and to consider their application to the care we provide.

How are your continuing professional development needs fulfilled?

Learning is a continuous process. Initially, when you are training, you learn theories, the normal anatomy and physiology; on the wards you learn the practical skills and practicalities behind disease processes and treatments. A sound knowledge base will allow you to understand why your patients need certain tests or medications. When you qualify, you have to put all the pieces together and think of the patient holistically, not just as a disease.

Nursing Times and *Nursing Standard* cover a wide range of topics and are easily read. There are hundreds of nursing publications covering every specialty imaginable so, once you have chosen an area or specialty, you can read a more comprehensive journal concentrating on the issues and practicalities affecting you and your patients.

A wide range of courses are available for continuing professional development depending on your chosen specialty. The ones most applicable across the specialties will be the annual updates from your Trust, often including cardio-pulmonary resuscitation (CPR), fire training and manual handling. Ward managers or team leaders carry out an annual appraisal to identify the development goals and knowledge needs that you require. A plan is formulated to help you to meet them.

How do you manage the conflicting demands of working with service users, colleagues and managers?

Nursing can be a difficult job on the best of days. The nature of the work requires that you will interact with many different people on any given day. There are therefore numerous opportunities for conflicting demands.

Conflicting demands can include trying to do the best for your patient while dealing with time constraints, a large workload and high expectations from senior staff. Good team work is essential in these cases. It is easy for one person to become overwhelmed, which reduces their effectiveness and affects their well-being. It is important to maintain communication with colleagues even when everyone is busy. I try to make sure that I always get a break even when there are still things to do (there will always be something to do!). By making sure that I am not hungry or dehydrated I can work more effectively.

Sometimes I may have to emphasise to next of kin that the patient is my main priority. It is important not to enter into family feuds or arguments and to always strive for a healthy environment in which the patient can recover. Illegal or immoral behaviour by patients, family members or visitors should not be tolerated. Most hospitals now have a zero tolerance policy where individuals persisting in antisocial behaviour can be ejected from the hospital and, in extreme cases, banned from the hospital. This might include drug taking, violence and abusive behaviour to staff, other patients or family members. Thirteen per cent of National Health Service staff have experienced violence in their working environment (Healthcare Commission, 2007).

Professional conflicts in the workplace can range from not entering into inappropriate relationships with patients to suspecting that a colleague is unfit to practise due to drug or alcohol problems. In any case always know whom to confide in, be it your ward sister or ward manager, as they will know what action to take and will support you in any way required.

Key learning points

- Nursing is a demanding but rewarding career.
- Support is available to help with difficult situations.
- As a patient's nurse, you are expected to protect the patient when vulnerable, ensure their safety, facilitate them getting the information or support that they may need and speak up for the patient if they are not able to do so for themselves.
- Ethical issues are part of everyday work.
- Team work is crucial for both patient and nurse well-being.

REFLECTION ACTIVITIES

1. You have a patient who does not speak English. How will this affect your use of interpersonal skills?
2. After a prolonged resuscitation attempt on a patient, a colleague appears very upset and you worry that it may affect their work. How might you discuss this with them?

FURTHER READING

Beauchamp, T. and Childress, J. (2001) *Principles of Biomedical Ethics* (5th Ed.). New York: Oxford University Press

Bush, K. (2001) 'Are you really listening to your patient?' *Registered Nurse*, 64(3): 35–7

Egan, G. (1998) *The Skilled Helper*. Chichester: Wiley

Richards, A. and Edwards, S. (2003) *A Nurse's Survival Guide to the Ward*. Edinburgh: Churchill Livingstone

Chapter 8

Interpersonal Skills in Midwifery

Jenny Edwins

EDITOR'S INTRODUCTION

In this chapter Jenny introduces some aspects of the role of a practising midwife in a number of settings. She illustrates the complexity and diversity of experiences and emphasises the key skill of communication that underpins every interaction, enabling midwives to communicate effectively and meaningfully with women and their families.

Tennant and Butler (2007) identify communication and relationships as central and defining features of a 'good' midwife and Jenny's chapter explores all aspects of these features and their value to the women that midwives support.

In common with Lisa Collicott (Chapter 7), Jenny's role as a midwife requires that she is able to form relationships with women, sometimes in a very short period of time.

Key themes

- Reflection.
- Diversity.
- Supervision.
- Evidence-based practice.

Pre-reading reflection activity

In 2005 the International Confederation of Midwives (ICM) gave a definition of the term 'midwife'. Read it at **www. internationalmidwives.org/Portals/5/Documentation/ ICM%20Definition%20of%20the%20Midwife%202005.pdf** It identifies the range of responsibilities of the modern midwife and will provide a foundation for Jenny's more detailed discussion of the role.

JENNY EDWINS – MIDWIFE

Describe the kind of interactions that you might have with people in the course of a normal working day

The role of the midwife is incredibly diverse. Public perceptions usually focus upon the idea of the midwife as a person who 'delivers' babies but their remit is much wider than that. Maternity services have developed over time in response to major government reports and the newly qualified midwife of today is a highly skilled practitioner at the point of registration who must be 'fit for practice'. This means that they have to have the ability to care for women safely throughout pregnancy, labour and the post-natal period, extending up to 28 days after the birth of the baby. Recent publications from the Department of Health that are currently driving the ways in which midwives work include the *National Service Framework for Children, Young People and the Maternity Services* (DoH, 2004a) and the *Maternity Matters* report (DoH/Partnerships for Children, Families and Maternity, 2007). Both of these publications emphasise the need to deliver services that are tailored to the individual woman and her family, identifying the need for working in partnership with service users. Innovations that can improve access to maternity services and focus upon public health are being encouraged, but the fundamental delivery of care currently remains split into the two areas of community practice and hospital services. Some midwives work in the private sector and a very small number work independently.

A midwife working in the community has the opportunity to build **therapeutic** relationships with women over a period of time. As soon as a woman has had a positive pregnancy test she can access a midwife at an antenatal clinic to initiate a referral into the system of care. Midwives' clinics might be located in a GP practice, health centre or, increasingly, in children's centres.

Once a woman's pregnancy has been identified, an appointment will be made for the community midwife to visit her at home and undertake a detailed assessment known as 'booking'. Because the woman is in her own environment it should be easier to establish a more equal relationship with the professional, who is a guest. The booking visit takes a considerable amount of time as the midwife has to collect and share a lot of information. This will include obstetric, medical and social histories and a great deal of time is taken to discuss options for screening for conditions such as HIV (human immunodeficiency virus) and Down's syndrome. The overall aim of this assessment is to identify whether or not a woman will require referral to a hospital consultant for more intensive antenatal care. This will occur if any risk factors are identified at the booking visit. Women whose pregnancies are low risk will continue to be cared for in the community by the midwife. Low-risk women generally enjoy continuity of care from the same community midwife. They will meet at antenatal clinics throughout the pregnancy and care from that same midwife continues after the birth of the baby. Women who choose a home birth may also have a known community midwife caring for them in labour.

Antenatal and postnatal care encompasses many aspects linking into public health. In a normal working day a community midwife will draw upon their communication skills to build an effective relationship and this will often lead to the identification of particular needs or the disclosure of problems, such as living with domestic abuse. Midwives also have a statutory duty to act if they have concerns about child protection. If complex circumstances are identified it is the midwife's responsibility to refer the woman to the appropriate agency. Multidisciplinary working is vital because long-term specialist support may be needed that is outside of the scope of practice of a midwife. Tailored support or intervention might enable women with a need for specialist support, such as drug dependency or learning difficulties, to care for their baby and keep the family together. The new children's centres have the potential to improve multidisciplinary working and the introduction of the Common Assessment Framework (CAF) (DfES, 2006) is a tool that can be used by a number of health and social care professionals to aid effective communication.

Community midwives clearly have great opportunities to establish equal relationships with women over an extended period of time. When you speak to some women they will tell you that they were quite sad when the midwife stopped visiting them because they had begun to view them as a friend.

Maternity Matters (DoH/Partnerships for Children, Families and Maternity, 2007) states that by the end of 2009 women will have a number of 'choice guarantees' to enable them to make informed choices about their plan of care. One of these choice guarantees relates to the place of birth. The options for place of birth are:

- birth supported by a midwife at home;
- birth supported by a midwife in a local midwifery facility such as a designated local midwifery unit or birth centre – the unit might be based in the community or in a hospital; patterns of care vary across the country to reflect different local needs. These units promote a philosophy of normal and natural labour and childbirth;
- birth supported by a maternity team in a hospital. The team may include midwives, obstetricians, paediatricians and anaesthetists. For some women, this type of care will be the safest option but they too should have a choice of hospital.

(DoH/Partnerships for Children, Families and Maternity, 2007, pp. 12–13)

Midwives are present at the great majority of births. Birth centres are often described as 'free standing' and these units are generally staffed by midwives who have a base or link with community services. Midwife-led units are generally sited adjacent to a consultant unit. If the chosen place of birth is a consultant unit it is unlikely that a woman will have previously met the midwife caring for her during labour. A positive and trusting relationship therefore has to be facilitated at a time when women are extremely vulnerable and heavily reliant upon the support of the midwife and their ability to establish a trusting and effective channel of communication in a very short space of time.

After an uncomplicated birth a woman and her baby may leave the delivery suite and return home or they may choose to spend a short period of time in a postnatal ward. This postnatal hospital stay is extended for those women and babies who have had more complex births, including those who are recovering from a caesarean section. The level of care at this time can therefore be quite intense and a woman who has had major surgery to birth her baby will initially need a degree of nursing care and a lot of support to establish breast feeding, if that is her choice.

Effective midwifery care after a complicated birth requires great sensitivity. Psychological needs can be immense if a woman is separated from her baby who has been admitted to a special care or neonatal intensive care unit. There are also extremely sad occasions when a baby dies around the time of birth and this situation will be very demanding for all of the staff concerned with the woman's care. Caring for bereaved parents requires special skills that exercise a great deal of sensitivity and many units have designated specialist 'bereavement midwife' posts to support women and staff in the most appropriate way.

What are the key skills that you use in your work with people?

Communication

Maternity care underwent a virtual revolution in the 1990s with the publication of the *Changing Childbirth* report (DoH, 1993). The main message of this report was encapsulated within the ethos of placing women at the centre of care. The three 'Cs' of Choice, Continuity and Control launched the concept of partnership working, aiming to truly involve service users at every stage as active participants in their own plan of care. It is clear that excellent communication skills are vital if this is the aim and the ability of a midwife to listen actively is undeniably crucial.

Childbearing is a life-changing event and the experience is highly individual. Rogers (1978) describes the theory of **unconditional positive regard** that offers a framework, based in counselling theory, which prompts practitioners from all disciplines to adopt an open approach that views any individual without prejudice or assumption. A professional in a position of power can be influenced by others in their initial assessment of a woman's needs or lifestyle. It is all too easy to draw stereotypical assumptions and the following case study might help to illustrate this point.

Case study

In a busy consultant maternity unit there is generally an established ritual at the changeover of shifts when staff teams meet collectively to review the care of all women on the delivery suite and exchange important information relating to the care of each woman in labour. There is an imperative to conduct this handover of care in a professional and comprehensive manner and the following true account is distressing in the fact that this might

---

not always be assured. In fact, it is an excellent example of how not to do it.

An unsupported 17-year-old woman was in labour and this was progressing normally. Her low-risk status did not offer any cause for concern. The midwife handing over her care remarked at some length upon the fact that the woman had a distinctive tattoo on the inner aspect of one of her thighs. The tattoo consisted of a suggestive statement of an explicit sexual nature. As a result, a picture of this young woman was conveyed to the incoming team of midwives of a young person who was unintentionally pregnant because of her immoral behaviour and inconsistent lifestyle.

The attitude of the midwife handing over the care of this woman was inexcusable. As the woman's advocate the midwife should have acted professionally in handing over her care without drawing any inference or stereotypical conclusions. Young women are often disproportionately at risk due to their social circumstances and, as a result, they are over-represented in the statistics relating to maternal deaths (Lewis, 2004). If the midwife had used the skill of active listening to establish an equal relationship with the woman, she might have identified a vulnerable individual who needed a great deal of support. There may also have been unrecognised needs for ongoing support after the birth of the baby that required referral to initiate multi-agency support.

In reality, the majority of midwives that I have had the privilege to work with have excellent communication skills and the above case study is definitely not typical.

Women in labour are experiencing a phenomenally powerful event. They can have expectations that are unfulfilled and this is clearly the case when a planned home birth does not happen and the woman has to be transferred into hospital because of complications. A woman-centred approach that acknowledges the emotional component of such a situation is illustrated in the next case study.

Case study

B had planned to give birth to her first baby at home. She was a healthy 30-year-old woman who had no reason to anticipate that she could not birth her baby without any intervention. Labour began normally but, after many hours of coping with strong contractions at home, it became clear that a spontaneous birth was not going to happen. The community midwife caring for B arranged for transfer to hospital and I was the midwife allocated to take over her care when she arrived on the labour ward.

B was upset at the turn of events but had not 'given up'. I listened to her closely when we met, rather than talking to her. B told me that she was feeling very tired because she had been trying to push her baby out at home for over an hour. She asked for an epidural and this request was met so that she could rest for a while. Once the epidural became effective we had the opportunity to discuss what had happened so far and what might happen next. B was still keen to try to push her baby out herself and we made a plan to start the pushing process again and to reassess the situation within a stated period of time if the birth was not imminent. We seemed to build up a rapport very easily and the feeling in the room was positive despite the disappointment that B had felt at having to come into hospital to have her baby.

After pushing for a period of time it was clear to me that the baby was not going to be born vaginally. I shared my observation that, despite B's excellent pushing efforts, the baby had not moved any further down the birth canal. B was naturally disappointed, but agreed that it was now time to ask the obstetrician to review her options. We subsequently went calmly into theatre and the baby was born by caesarean section.

A planned home birth was what B had wanted but she had few regrets after the operation. She felt as though she had seized the opportunity to give birth at home – it hadn't gone to plan but she was consulted in relation to the decision to come into hospital and had tried her very best to push the baby out under her own steam. The need for a caesarean section was clear to B because she had exhausted all other avenues.

When I think back upon caring for B I feel that I did well in supporting her through a difficult birth. 'Support' is a word used very liberally in relation to the role of the midwife but it is quite difficult to define what 'support' is. Another term used frequently is 'empowerment'. I believe that I supported B sensitively during the later stages of her labour by using my skill of active listening to understand how she was feeling and coping with the fact that her plans had not materialised. This allowed me to empathise with her situation and to identify her need for detailed information about her progress. I was also very honest and open in sharing my professional opinions. Both mother and baby were healthy at the end of the experience. B subsequently made a smooth transition to motherhood, despite her unrealised home birth, because she was fully informed and involved in the decisions regarding her care. It could also be said that she was enabled, or empowered, to do so because of the effective midwifery support that she received around the time of the birth of her baby.

There are some occasions when a midwife cannot use active listening skills in order to build a relationship with women in the conventional way. It can be challenging to care for women in labour when you do not share a common language and non-verbal skills have to be relied upon. Interpreter services are readily available in some areas of the UK but many areas are poorly served. The cost of interpreters can be an issue that limits access to a great extent and there are many problems in relying upon family members to act as interpreters.

Listening to and interpreting the sounds that a woman makes as her labour progresses are traditional cues that inform midwives about the progress of labour, but it may take some experience before a midwife is confident enough to feel acutely attuned to these signals and to rely on them totally. These cues will provide the midwife with a wealth of information about the physiological processes driving the woman's labour but the midwife still needs to find a way to communicate with the woman in order to support her effectively.

Case study

Mrs B was admitted to the labour ward because her pregnancy was prolonged and her consultant had advised induction of labour. Mr B was accompanying his wife – he spoke some English but was not fluent. The prescribed procedure for induction of labour was documented in the case notes as artificial rupture

▶

of the membranes (breaking the bag of waters in front of the baby's head). This is an invasive procedure involving a vaginal examination. It stimulates contractions but carries some risks, so it is very important to obtain a woman's consent before carrying out this intervention. The consultant had talked to the couple in the antenatal clinic prior to Mrs B's admission but the midwife caring for them was not happy to proceed with the induction. She felt that the couple's understanding of the implications of the procedure was inadequate because of the language barrier. Interpreter services in this unit were scarce so the midwife rang the hospital switchboard to ask whether there was any member of the medical staff on duty who spoke the couple's language. Fortunately, there was a doctor who was willing and able to come to the labour ward to act as an interpreter and assist in obtaining the woman's informed consent. This interaction was documented but, once the interpreter left the labour ward, the midwife had to continue caring for the woman using non-verbal communication skills. Artificial rupture of the membranes initiated strong contractions and Mrs B went into labour very quickly. This can be an overwhelming experience for women and the midwife made sure that she was a constant physical presence for the woman by remaining in the room at all times.

There is evidence that continual support from a midwife during labour is beneficial for women and improves birth outcomes (Hodnett *et al.*, 2002). I am unaware of any specific research that informs practice when caring for women where midwives cannot communicate through a shared language, but logic dictates that a continual presence must be reassuring. The midwife could not offer any reassuring verbal explanation about the effects of the artificial rupture of the membranes as the contractions increased in strength. She could, however, maintain her supportive presence through appropriate means such as maintaining good eye contact, using a reassuring tone of voice (albeit in a foreign language), and appropriate touch by rubbing the woman's lower back at the height of each contraction. Tone of voice is particularly important because it can convey how a professional is feeling about the progress of labour. Women need to feel safe if their labour hormones are going to work effectively and a calm voice gives the message that all is well. Another point that may seem obvious, is that raising your voice and speaking loudly will not enable anybody to understand you if you do not share a common language.

Mrs B's labour progressed very quickly. Most women find that the intensity of the sensations associated with advanced labour and birth are difficult to cope with. Women often cope with these strong sensations through vocalising loudly and following their instincts, adopting positions dictated by nature to give birth spontaneously. Words are often superfluous at this point but the midwife supported Mrs B by talking quietly in a soothing and reassuring manner, aiming to reassure her that all was progressing normally. As soon as the baby was born and in Mrs B's arms the midwife knew that she had supported Mrs B effectively when she looked directly at the midwife and smiled, while squeezing her hand strongly to say 'thank you'.

Supporting women and their partners psychologically

The time around birth is usually a straightforward and happy event. Midwives are referred to as 'guardians of normal birth' and, in my opinion, this might be because there is nothing more satisfying than supporting a woman to give birth to her baby and acknowledging that our bodies are remarkable. But sometimes pregnancy, birth or the postnatal period become complicated and the midwife has to identify these problems, act appropriately and support the woman and her family at a very difficult and anxiety-provoking time.

Case study

S was in labour with her second baby and ready to give birth. The baby's head was born slowly and the midwife had to help to ease its chin out. When the baby did not turn to deliver its shoulder, the midwife realised that there was a problem and I answered the call bell to go and help her. This was an acute emergency and an urgent call was sent out for medical assistance. In the meantime, I introduced myself hastily to the couple and then used a number of manoeuvres to deliver the baby. I had to manipulate the position of the baby to release her trapped shoulder by placing my fingers on the back of the other shoulder to push it into a better position. When this did not work I placed my fingers in front of the shoulder to push it in the other direction. This worked immediately and the baby was born shortly after – but she wasn't breathing because of the delay in the birth process. A paediatrician arrived and the baby responded well as she was resuscitated.

It is very important to acknowledge that parents can be deeply traumatised by a difficult birth and, as the baby began to respond, I communicated with the parents to tell them that she was doing well. It is important to be truthful in situations like this. It would be wrong to give false reassurances so it is advisable to stick to the facts: 'your baby is breathing well now – her colour is pink and that's really good – you should be able to hold her soon'.

When I think back to this birth I can remember being totally focused on the procedures I had to carry out. I had rehearsed them many times at training sessions and often in my head. In a way it was as if I was on auto pilot and the other midwife did a great job in supporting the couple at that time. It was only after the baby was seen to be healthy and crying that I had time to communicate properly with the parents. It was important to give them time to talk about why I had acted as I did, so that they had a clear understanding of what happened during the birth. The husband told me that he had been terrified and had felt like pushing me out of the way to pull the baby out forcefully himself. I acknowledged that he must have been extremely frightened and explained exactly what I had done. The baby had small bruises behind and in front of her shoulders from the imprints of my fingers where I had exerted the pressure to turn them. The paediatrician offered reassurance to the parents that this was not a problem and that the baby would be fine. I think that it was vital to talk the parents through what had happened so that they could make sense of it. I feel that I did this well and I can support this statement because when S had her third baby, a few years later, I met her in the postnatal ward and she and her husband were very pleased to see me again. And I was delighted to meet the baby (who was now a lively toddler) that I had helped to deliver in those difficult circumstances.

If the psychological needs of parents are not met there can be repercussions, both in relation to women's mental health and the dynamics of the family unit. It is strongly suggested, but not actually proven, that traumatic events around birth are linked with postnatal depression and post traumatic stress disorder (Snow, 2008). Good midwifery care identifies that women are individuals and have a range of needs. This approach is often referred to as 'holism'. Holism identifies that it is inappropriate to compartmentalise aspects of care because we all have physical, psychosocial and spiritual needs that need to be met to live a fulfilling and healthy life (Jones, 1998).

The ability of a midwife to make appropriate evidence-based decisions in critical situations that may compromise women's physical and psychological health is tested on a daily basis. There is always an opportunity to learn from reflecting on our experiences and it is a key component of training to be a midwife. We can learn more about midwifery practice every day through the process of reflection and after qualification this must be continued to demonstrate life-long learning, the result of which will improve the quality of midwifery interactions with women over time.

Which theoretical frameworks underpin your practice?

Earlier in this chapter I mentioned that midwifery care should be centred upon the needs of women and their families. Roger's (1978) philosophy of unconditional positive regard can be a good starting point if it is adopted because it identifies that all individuals have their own valid perspectives and the free will to exercise choice. This offers a foundation to build equal relationships where the woman is a partner in planning her care, rather than a passive recipient who accepts that professionals automatically know best what is right for her and her baby.

An equal partnership in care means that the midwife must effectively share evidence-based information to equip women with a clear basis to make informed decisions for themselves. Models with their roots in counselling can be useful to give professionals a framework to work within, but it has to be remembered that midwives are not trained counsellors who are aiming to help individuals to work through complex long-standing problems. However, as a professional group, midwives need to develop particular counselling skills. One framework that I have found useful and easy to use is Heron's (1990) six-category intervention analysis model. It identifies helpful interventions, or actions, that aim to facilitate decision-making. The first three interventions fall into an authoritative style and include information giving and challenging. The remainder can be classified as the counselling skills of supporting, drawing out and allowing emotional release. All of Heron's interventions are dependent on good communication skills, the most important being active listening.

Pairman (2000) studied the nature of the relationship between women and their midwives in New Zealand to identify the theory that many women view it as a 'professional friendship'. She describes how real friendships are generally spontaneous but the midwife and the woman will only form a partnership because of the pregnancy. The partnership between a woman and her midwife is unique in that it is time limited within clear boundaries, despite its intimate nature. If the midwife has done a good job in supporting the woman throughout the childbearing experience, as a professional friend, the relationship will come to a natural end as the woman confidently carries on into motherhood.

What is the legislative framework that underpins your practice?

The Nursing and Midwifery Council (NMC) regulates midwifery practice and their main objective is to protect the public. They regularly review the quality of midwifery education to make sure that student midwives have every opportunity to become competent practitioners. At the point of qualification a midwife is entered onto the register and allocated a personal identification number (PIN). This allows employers to check that a midwife applying for a job has a valid qualification. There is also a yearly requirement for midwives to register their intention to practise in a specified location and a three-yearly requirement for each individual registrant to demonstrate that they have updated their practice.

The NMC produces professional guidelines and standards to support midwifery practice and assure high standards of care for the public. Some of the publications are generic such as *The Code: Standards of Conduct, Performance and Ethics for Nurses and Midwives* (NMC, 2008a) and the *Standards for Medicines Management* (NMC, 2008b). The most prominent guide specific to midwifery is the *Midwives Rules and Standards* (NMC, 2004a), which includes clear definitions of a midwife's responsibilities and sphere of practice.

Midwifery is unique in maintaining an additional system of statutory supervision that has the clear remit of protecting the public.

Statutory supervision of midwives has operated in the UK for over 100 years. It has developed to become a means by which midwives are supported in, and with, their practice. As a modern regulatory practice, statutory supervision of midwives supports protection of the public by:

- promoting best practice and excellence in care
- preventing poor practice and
- intervening in unacceptable practice.

(NMC, 2006a)

Experienced midwives can opt to undertake additional training to become a supervisor of midwives (SOM) and every midwife should have an annual review with their nominated SOM. This is an opportunity to explore ways in which a midwife's professional development can be enhanced. SOMs are also available to offer advice and support in relation to complex practice issues and, if the midwife is involved in a case where the outcome has been poor, the SOM will offer ongoing support.

What are the ethical issues that impact on your practice?

Pregnancy and birth are life-changing events that encompass numerous ethical issues. Midwives are compelled to work within an ethical and legal framework that acknowledges the right of each woman to exercise her autonomy. This means that any mentally competent individual has the freedom to make decisions about her care, even when that decision is contrary to any medical advice. The role of the midwife lies in ensuring that the woman has been able to access evidence-based information to inform her decision. Once the woman has made her decision the midwife has a duty of care to continue the provision of a high standard of midwifery care.

Case study

L was in her late twenties and pregnant with her fifth baby. She had accepted a screening blood test to assess the risk of her baby having Down's syndrome and the result of this test indicated that the risk was very high. The next step involved an amniocentesis. This is a procedure where a fine needle is inserted into the woman's abdomen in order to take a sample of the amniotic fluid surrounding the baby. The chromosomes of the baby are then examined to ascertain whether or not there is an extra chromosome 21, the presence of which is diagnostic of Down's syndrome.

As L's community midwife I worked closely with her consultant obstetrician and when the result of the amniocentesis was found to be positive he asked me to visit her at home to give the result to her.

Screening tests exist to identify specific conditions that are treatable in order to minimise the impact of the condition and maximise health. Screening for Down's syndrome is an anomaly in this context, as there is no treatment for the condition. Termination of pregnancy is the current medical 'solution' after diagnosis of the condition and this is a huge ethical and legal issue in itself that will not be explored here. After discovering

▶

---

that her baby had a diagnosis of Down's syndrome, and taking some time to consider the implications, L decided to continue her pregnancy. Baby P was born at term and welcomed into the family. As L's midwife I learnt a great deal about how easy it is to presume that women will make the choice that professionals deem to be appropriate and I subsequently carried out a research project to explore the reasons why women might choose to continue their pregnancy in such a situation (Edwins, 2008). My role in supporting L throughout her pregnancy and the early days of parenting were a continuation of the care that any community midwife could provide, but it was very important to ensure that the health visitor and general practitioner were fully involved to ensure that plans were in place for the continuing care of the baby and the family as a whole.

L's story illustrates just one ethical issue that a midwife might meet in practice. In midwifery practice there are ethical issues to be addressed every day and decision-making is also guided by law. The two issues of ethics and law are nearly always linked. Where situations are complex a midwife can seek advice from a manager, supervisors of midwives, professional organisation or NHS Trust legal department.

Working with people can be very demanding. How do you care for yourself?

Midwifery is undeniably a very demanding profession in both a physical and psychological sense. Most midwives based in a hospital environment work a shift pattern that is antisocial and physically taxing. There is often a requirement to rotate through a system of day and night duty within a short space of time and this can take its toll upon a midwife's health. Community midwives participate in an 'on call' system for emergencies and home births and this means that they may be expected to work all night following a full day at work. These are clearly factors that might impinge on family life and a great number of midwives are resolving this work/home life imbalance by choosing to work part-time hours. The number of midwives now working part time has had an impact on staffing levels and there is currently a shortage of midwives in many areas. This has increased the workload and is a significant stressor in many maternity units. The workforce is under review and there has to be an increase in midwife numbers in the near future if the pledges made in the *Maternity Matters* document (DoH/Partnerships for Children, Families and Maternity, 2007) are going to be realised. Until that time, midwives continue to manage their psychological health, in general, through peer support and informal debriefing, or through accessing the system of midwifery supervision, when difficulties or poor outcomes occur. Most NHS trusts have counselling services available should staff need further or ongoing psychological support.

Key learning points

- Midwives need to be able to communicate effectively with women and their families.
- Midwives promote health and well-being.
- Sometimes there can be difficulties or poor outcomes for women and their babies.
- Midwives work within a statutory framework that defines their scope of practice.
- There is a need to work in partnership with other health professionals or agencies when women present with complex needs.

REFLECTION ACTIVITIES

1. Visit the website of the largest professional organisation for midwives in the UK at **www.rcm.org.uk** to identify the range of activities that midwifery practice encompasses and the opportunities that exist for professional development.
2. Consider the skills and sensitivity that practising midwives need to support parents when a baby dies. Visit the SANDS (Stillbirth and Neonatal Death Society) website at **www.uk-sands.org** to gain an insight into the needs of bereaved families.
3. The public health role of the midwife is growing and improving breast feeding rates is a priority for the health of the nation. Find out more about a global initiative called the 'Baby Friendly Initiative' at **www. babyfriendly.org.uk** and identify the considerable range of related skills in which midwives have to be up to date.

FURTHER READING

Edwins, J. (2008) *Community Midwifery Practice*. Oxford: Blackwell Science

Frith, L. and Draper, H. (2003) *Ethics and Midwifery: Issues in Contemporary Practice*. Hale: Books for Midwives Press

International Confederation of Midwives (2005) 'Definition of the Midwife'. Online at: **www.internationalmidwives.org/Portals/5/ Documentation/ICM%20Definition%20of%20the%20Midwife%20 2005.pdf** (accessed 6 August 2007)

Leap, N. and Hunter, B. (1993) *The Midwife's Tale: An Oral History from Handywoman to Professional Midwife*. London: Scarlet Press

Wickham, S. (2003–6), *Midwifery: Best Practice*, Vol 1–4. Hale: Books for Midwives Press

Useful websites

Midwifery Network online – a network for midwives, student midwives and those who want to enter midwifery: **www.midwiferynetwork. com**

Midwifery Taster Day – an award winning innovation for those thinking about midwifery training: **www.worcester.ac.uk/courses/3013.html**

The Royal College of Midwives – professional organisation with up to date information about numerous aspects of midwifery: **www.rcm. org.uk**

Chapter 9

Interpersonal Skills in General Practice

Dr Andrew Chapman

EDITOR'S INTRODUCTION

In this chapter you will learn about some of the ways in which GPs use interpersonal skills with their patients. GPs are the first point of contact that most of us have with the National Health Service (NHS) and, as such, our interactions with them may well define our view of all health professionals.

Key themes

- Interdisciplinary working.
- Continuing professional development.
- Professional responsibility.

Pre-reading reflection activity

To gain another perspective of the working life of a GP read an extract from D. Haslam (2003) 'A day in the life of a GP . . .' which you can find at **www.gprecruitment.org.uk/gpcareers/life.htm**

ANDREW CHAPMAN – GP

GPs undergo a limited apprenticeship in hospital medicine before finding themselves in the place where it is likely that they will remain for the rest of their career, a period of between 25 and 35 years. The patients that they see will not be sorted into speciality but will be defined by their geographical locality, usually the same locality as is occupied by the doctor. In general practice there is no hierarchy, even the concept of Senior Partner is nothing more than an indication that one individual has been around longer than the others. The career of a GP is **longitudinal** by which I mean that the kind of work undertaken and the type of patient seen on the first day of their career as a GP will be exactly the same as that which they will experience on the day that they retire.

The case study below encapsulates many of the issues about being a doctor and, in particular, about being a general practitioner. Not that all consultations deal with such serious disease or such far-reaching issues as those in this case study. It is a universal characteristic of general practice that it is quite unpredictable. There are consultations about trivial matters, self-limiting disease that is uncomfortable but not life-threatening, but there are never trivial consultations. The truth of this is to be found in an important characteristic of general practice, its longitudinal nature.

Case study

I had known Harold as a patient since I'd come to the area. I found him to be a difficult man to get along with. He was a successful local businessman and district councillor, but I found him overbearing. To start with he had tried to bully me. He got nowhere with that, but I suspected that he bullied his wife, Katherine.

Harold had once been a big man. He was broad-shouldered and full of confidence. Cancer had reduced him to a sack of angular bones, contained by his brownish-yellow skin. His eyes were sunk in his head, his cheeks pulled in. His larynx was so prominent that you could see all its anatomical features. His breath was raspy and impeded as if he would have preferred not to breathe at all but knew that he had to keep it going. The cancer was killing him. The pain was severe.

Katherine was a soft-spoken woman who always dressed well. She appeared in awe of her husband. I found that I got on much better with her than I did with Harold. It was she who spoke to me first about her husband's illness.

'I am worried about him, Doctor. He seems to be getting more and more pain in his tummy. He says it's indigestion but I don't think so. He won't come and see you, says it would be a waste of time, not that I mean you would waste his time.' She seemed flustered. 'It's all right, Katherine. I know what you mean.' I paused to think. 'Why don't you tell him that you've spoken to me and that I would be happy to see him?' Behind this conversation I could feel his fear, almost tangible. 'Sometimes people change their minds if they know there is someone to help.'

She did try it and Harold eventually came to see me. As I listened to his story I was pretty certain what the trouble was. Before I examined him I said: 'What have you been telling yourself about this pain?' I kept my gaze on his face. What I saw was incomprehension shortly followed by fear, then bluster and aggression.

'Nothing at all, doctor. I thought it was your job to work that out.'

'Nothing at all?' I said, still keeping my gaze on his face.

'Oh, dammit, man. Yes, of course I've been telling myself things. Telling myself it must be OK, it can't be serious.' There was the briefest of pauses before he continued: 'I don't convince myself, though.' Now he looked at me and the fear was obvious.

Not letting my gaze drop I said, as gently as I could, 'Let's have a look at you then.' Touching could stand in for words. Harold undressed and lay on the examination couch. I put my hand on his abdomen. There was no difficulty in feeling the hard, craggy mass just below the rib cage on the left side but I was careful to examine the rest of him with as much attention. I needed to signal at this early stage in his illness that he would be taken seriously, treated with care, treated as a man with an illness, not a lump in a patient. As he dressed I went to fetch Katherine. The three of us sat together in a triangle of concern.

'Well Harold, I can detect a mass in your tummy.' He cut in.

'Mass, doctor. What sort of mass?'

▶

'It feels like a tumour, probably on your bowel. You will have to have further investigations but I am afraid that it looks as if it is cancer.'

Bald, unmodified fact. No euphemisms at this point. Silence for a few moments. Harold whistled 'Strewth! I never thought it would be that. What does this mean, doc? Will I have to have an operation?'

'Quite probably', I answered, 'but first it must be confirmed. I would like to refer you to Mr Curwen. He is a very experienced surgeon.'

'Let's get on with it then, doctor. I'll see him privately, of course.' I had expected nothing different. After the necessary arrangements had been made they left. Harold stood up, then turned and held out his hand and said, 'Thanks Doc. It can't be easy for you.'

(Adapted from A. J. Chapman, 'Beyond the Silence' (unpublished).)

In the case study above the GP talks about knowing his patient in his role in the community. Doctors are enmeshed in the community in which they live but there is a sense in which they are, at the same time, separate from their socio-cultural environment: outsiders yet within. One of the points that I am trying to make here is that every episodic encounter with a patient adds something to the longitudinal relationship with that patient, whether positive or negative. In the consultation about a sore throat the doctor may recognise trivial illness but the consultation is part of a much longer, multifaceted relationship between patient and doctor. It is never trivial.

Describe the kind of interactions that you might have with people in the course of a normal working day

In any one day a doctor may see between 20 and 50 patients (in some cases many more). The time allocation for each consultation seems to have settled at around ten minutes. This bald fact has always had the capacity to horrify me. What on earth can be achieved in so short a time? Counsellors and therapists have their protected hour; how can GPs pretend to do anything effective within a ten-minute span? However, they do and part of the reason is the longitudinal aspect of their work. When the patient comes into the consulting room a relationship already exists, frequently alluded to in the dictum, 'GPs know their patients'. That statement is true but what may be more important is the parallel assertion, 'patients know their doctor'. In that latter case 'knowing' is something akin to ownership – people refer to 'my doctor'. Thus each consultation does not start from square one; it carries with it a past, a present and a future. Truly longitudinal.

So far we have considered consultations in which there is clear, recognisable disease. There are many consultations where the presence or absence of physical disease is clear (and from here on I shall use the term 'disease' to mean physical disease, which contrasts with the term 'illness', which is a state experienced by a patient). There are many more consultations where the illness is diffuse and difficult to define. In order to understand the interactions that might take place in that brief ten minutes between doctor and patient it is necessary to move back in time, to consider the antecedents to the consultation.

It is reasonable to assert that the process starts when an individual undergoes a change in health. This change in health might be a pain felt in the left-hand side of chest that comes and goes. Or it might be a sleep disorder that has the individual waking each morning at 3 a.m. feeling wretched. Or it might be, like the first case study, a persistent abdominal pain. Studies have shown that very few symptoms (what we are calling 'changes in health') end up as consultations with a doctor, perhaps only 1 in 20. Let us consider what happens to the rest.

When an individual experiences a change in health the first thing that they are likely to do is to talk to themselves about it. Later we shall see how important this internal dialogue is. The individual may say: 'Why have I got this pain in my chest? It's probably chopping all those logs yesterday. It'll wear off.' That is one kind of response and assuming that time and rest allow the symptom to wear off the individual takes no further action (except, perhaps, to leave the log chopping to someone else). But suppose there had been no log chopping. The individual, perhaps a person prone to becoming anxious, might think: 'It's chest pain on my left. My heart is on my left, perhaps it's heart pain.'

This internal dialogue calls on a person's understanding of the position of the heart and the likelihood that heart pain is thus felt on the left side of the chest. Understandings like this, and there are many of them, are termed 'health beliefs'. We all have them even if we rarely speak of them. They may be soundly based on anatomical concepts but more often they are not. In this example, for instance, we know that the heart is, in fact, a central organ; it is rather more prominent on the left than on the right. Pain from the heart is felt centrally but this person's health beliefs tell her otherwise.

Patients may also continue this internal dialogue by asking themselves questions, such as 'what is the likelihood of my having so-and-so (heart disease, depression, etc.)?' Obviously, this draws on health beliefs once more but the application is in the field of prediction, like betting on the horses. Thus the individual who experiences chest pain may say to himself: 'My father died of a coronary at 57, my uncle has just had a coronary artery bypass, this could be serious.' Clearly he is likely to take things further. On the other hand another individual may say: 'There has never been any heart disease in my family and, in any case, I'm a woman and women are much less at risk of heart attacks than men. It was probably those logs.' She is not going to take things further, at least not at the moment.

There is yet another factor that affects help-seeking behaviour and that is expressed by the self-question: 'What is the cost if I do something about so-and-so?' Decisions are never made in a vacuum and the help-seeking individual is going to have some conception of what might happen if they continue down the road of seeking medical help. In some societies (mercifully not for us in the UK at the moment) there are real considerations of financial cost but there are also other determinants; investigations may be painful and unpleasant, time from work cannot be lost when there is a big contract on. The patient with the sleep disorder is quite well-informed; he recognises that his change of sleeping pattern may be depression. His mother was hospitalised by section for a similar illness and ended up dying by suicide. He himself does not want to admit that his illness may be similar. He keeps quiet about it.

There are many such ruminations when a change in health occurs. Some may lead the individual to speak to another person. This is likely to be a member of the family and the response may end things at that point, 'Don't you remember, you chopped all those logs yesterday? That's probably what did it.' Frequently the individual may speak to a member of the health professions – but not their own doctor. Midwives and district nurses are often asked, 'Should I take this to the doctor?' Note that the other person is not asked to diagnose, let alone treat. They are asked to help in the decision as to whether the individual should continue on the help-seeking path. Some people approach pharmacists, though how common this is, despite it being encouraged, is not fully known. Many people may also approach alternative medicine practitioners.

So, if the suffering individual makes it as far as having a consultation with his GP we can see that he is carrying much more than the symptom alone. He is likely to say, 'I have this pain in my chest', but we know that there is much more – fears, anxieties, probabilities, health beliefs and concerns as to what this is going to cost (in the broadest sense of the term). His doctor could choose to restrict her attention to the presenting symptom alone; she may be rushed, she may be tired, she may even dislike this man. But she knows well enough that all these covert considerations are there and will need skills to uncover them.

What are the key skills that you use in your work with people?

> Relationships based on openness, trust and good communication will enable the GP to work in partnership with patients to address their individual needs. (GMC, 2006)

Before I discuss the skills employed to achieve this task in what seems to be an impossibly short period of time, we need to look at what the doctor personally brings to the encounter. Firstly, the main concern of the doctor might be, 'Does this patient have a serious disease?' It is impossible to overemphasise the importance of this question. Just about every doctor experiences it. The expression used is 'to rule out' as in 'can I rule out cancer in this patient who complains of pain on the left side of the abdomen?' Some see the work of GPs as being 'to rule out', that is to exclude serious disease. Once that is done the patient can be despatched with bland reassurance. The trouble is that if that 'reassurance' does not address the patient's often unspoken concerns the consultation will not end satisfactorily. Nonetheless the possibility of serious disease is a major concern for the doctor.

So the modern doctor does not have great swathes of time in which to systematically explore their patient's problem. In any case the patient is likely to feel frustrated by being cross-questioned about their bowel function when what they really want to talk about is the fears that they have about their headaches. The newer skill that the doctor demonstrates is one of active listening. In the case study below the doctor uses two particular skills, the use of silence and the use of the 'what are you telling yourself about this?' question.

Case study

Doctor: 'Hello Patrick. Take a seat. How can I help you today?'
(Note the open question. It allows the patient to choose the agenda. 'What's wrong with you?' from the doctor would be too challenging and more likely to close the consultation down.)

Patrick: 'I'm not sure, doctor . . . it's these headaches. They've been coming every day for the last two weeks . . .' (At this point he seems to run out of steam. He sits still but the doctor notices that Patrick's hands are trembling. There is no difficulty in picking up the anxiety even though less than 20 words have been spoken. She says nothing. There is a silence for nearly half a minute.)

Now, at this point you may well be thinking that if there is so little time for this consultation, why is she wasting it sitting in silence? Should she not get on and ask some questions about those headaches? But let us explore what might be happening with each of them during this time when nothing is being said. As a doctor, familiar with this type of scenario, she has learnt over the years to empty her mind of possible questions, possible diagnoses. Instead she concentrates with close attention on what is in front of her, which is her patient, his symptom and the interaction between the two of them. At this point two things could happen. Patrick could end the silence:

Patrick (looking up): 'They're throbbing headaches, doctor.'

She will take particular note of what is said to end a silence. Such remarks are important. After all, unlike the doctor, Patrick has not been emptying his mind during the silence. He has been re-rehearsing all the thoughts, ideas and anxieties that brought him to the consultation in the first place, all those factors that we explored earlier. Her radar has picked up the word 'throbbing'. The fact that Patrick's headaches are experienced as throbbing has particular significance for him. The doctor's task is to unravel what is going on in his head apart from the headaches. She could interrogate him about his throbbing headaches. As we shall see later in this chapter this was the method used extensively in the past. But instead she asks one question, a very simple question (a similar question to one used in the extract at the start of this chapter).

> *Doctor*: 'What have you been telling yourself about these
>   throbbing headaches?' (A simple question but one with a
>   powerful effect. Sometimes it will provoke an angry response.)
> *Patrick*: 'I don't know. You're the doctor. You tell me!'(She does
>   not react to the anger but waits and, more often than not, she
>   will hear of the significance that the patient attaches to the
>   symptom.)
> *Patrick*: 'My mother had headaches. Throbbing ones. They called it
>   migraine until one day she had a brain haemorrhage and died.'
>   (Now the patient displays his vulnerability as he turns to face
>   the doctor.)
> *Patrick*: 'You don't think these headaches are the same, do you,
>   doctor?'
>
> This has cleared the air. Patient and doctor both acknowledge the
> anxiety. From here on it is a simple matter to determine the most
> likely cause of Patrick's headaches. She can even choose to explain
> the nature of his mother's haemorrhage, that it had no relationship
> to her migraine, that it was simply a chance association.

So Patrick leaves with appropriate medication for his headaches but, even more importantly, with a change in his health understanding. He has also contributed, with his doctor, in adding a building block to their relationship, a relationship that may stretch on for many years to come. Before he arrived he had one particular story that he told himself about himself. In the course of the brief ten-minute consultation he was enabled to modify that narrative to allow a small but significant shift in a story that he might, in future, find more comfortable to incorporate. Our lives are constructed of stories and no more so than in such stories of sickness. This is the creative work of healing. Doctor and patient, between them, are creating health.

It is given to doctors in our society to use a skill that is often denied to other therapists, the use of touch. In the first case study 'touching could stand in for words'. The touching of a patient, as part of a physical examination, can be both expressive and releasing. The way in which I, as a doctor, touch my patient can express concern, confidence, a willingness to take time, to take the patient seriously, even to calm anxiety. On occasions the crucial question or observation, the one that is emotionally laden, can be delayed until I am examining my patient, especially so when the patient is lying down (and thus vulnerable) and my hand is laid on their body rather than poking or prodding. The symbolism in the laying on of hands is very ancient and very powerful. As in any interaction between two people body language is very important. It behoves any doctor to be aware of what unspoken signals they are transmitting during the consultation. Writing notes or staring at a computer screen can be a serious disruption to the transaction between ill person and healer. Constant attentiveness is required of the doctor otherwise small signals, like the slightest flutter of the hand, the downturned gaze, may be missed. One particular phenomenon is important to catch, 'mirroring'. In this the patient and the doctor find themselves adopting the same posture and gestures as each other. It is a powerful signal for it usually indicates that there is significant empathy between the two. Sometimes the doctor can emulate mirroring and this can lead to a better communication between the two of them without anything being said.

It is important to re-emphasise that in the context of general practice the single consultation is but one building block among many in a continually developing therapeutic relationship. It is not as if that at each new consultation both participants start at square one. There may be much that has gone before, times when fear has been expressed and accepted, times when emotion has been shared, even times when challenges have been made.

Challenges can be useful but, badly handled, can act to the detriment of a useful patient–doctor relationship. The grossest of bad challenges, almost a caricature, is the 'pull yourself together' approach which is exemplified in the case study below.

Case study

Doctor: 'Come now, Mrs Smith, dozens of people have headaches. There is nothing seriously wrong with you, all the tests are normal.' (This is said in an attempt to bounce Mrs Smith out of the sick role that she is prone to adopt. It only requires the slightest of reflection to recognise that this is a covert angry response from a frustrated doctor, a situation we all find ourselves in from time to time.)

Challenges can be made in a different way. It is an approach that requires that the doctor can, as it were, stand back from the current discourse and observe what is going on, not just with his patient but also with himself. He can ask himself the question,

---

'what am I feeling at this exact moment?' The answer is important because the feeling that he identifies (and note he has not asked the question, 'what am I thinking?'; feelings are what he is after) is very likely to be the one that patient is feeling but is trying very hard to express. Here he has a way into the patient's psyche that he would be unlikely to find by simply asking. Once identified, the doctor can feed the feeling back. There are a number of ways to put it; one of the gentlest is to simply report what is happening.

Doctor: 'Mrs Smith, when you talk about your troubles with your daughter I feel quite sad.' (There is none of the confrontation of a direct question. Mrs Smith can make up her own mind as to whether she is going to respond; it is honest and truthful. It is very likely that it will produce a useful response.)

Mrs Smith (she has started to cry): 'I feel I've lost her, doctor. She's not the little girl I knew.'

The doctor's intervention has allowed this grief to be expressed. That grief might not have got through the barrier of anger and frustration that a mother feels about her aberrant daughter. The consultation can now continue at a deeper and more authentic level.

These are some of the ways that some doctors work for some of the time. The requirements of concentration can be very tiring. In these examples it could appear that to work in this way is always straightforward. The truth is that at times I am likely to feel totally at sea, at times the consultation does not run nearly as smoothly, often anger can surface and threaten to derail the process. Nonetheless this open, honest approach to meeting ill people always feels authentic.

What theoretical models underpin your practice?

Since the early twentieth century doctors, as medical students, have been taught a systematic approach to diagnosis (the task of detecting disease) known as 'clinical method'. For centuries before this the doctor's approach to ill patients was to make a detailed enquiry of the patient's symptoms, do hardly any physical examination and then diagnose by constructing an elaborate story to explain to the patient why they were experiencing the symptoms that they described. A physician's prowess depended mostly on the quality and conviction of these stories. This is an approach that is used by many alternative medicine practitioners to this day. Clinical method rebuilt this approach. It explored the history of the complaint, proceeded to a systematic questioning of all the bodily systems (cardiovascular, respiratory, etc.) and then undertook a general physical examination that included all the systems. In the case study at the beginning of this chapter you read how the doctor examining the mass in his patient's abdomen was 'careful to examine the rest of him with as much attention'. Naturally this approach is time-consuming. I used to use it when I was a house doctor in my first hospital job. Done properly it took at least 35 minutes. In fact it is a method that is rarely followed in full by practising doctors, be they consultants or GPs, but the underlying principle of systematic enquiry is lodged in our brains.

Many of these insights in this chapter come from psychoanalysis but it would be a mistake to regard this as some other kind of psychological treatment. This is about human beings talking about illness. Much that has been discussed here came from a series of seminars held by the psychoanalyst Michael Balint with a group of general practitioners in the 1950s. These took place over a period of ten years or so and spawned a number of publications. The most famous was the first, *The Doctor, His Patient and the Illness* (1957). It is widely regarded as being one of the most important texts that created modern general practice.

More recently the concept of story has been developed, the idea that we all tell stories about ourselves and our lives. Exploration of how stories can be affected by sickness is beautifully expounded by Brody (2002).

It remains important to recognise that general practice is an eclectic discipline and general practitioners are never happier than when working eclectically, acquiring skills and developing insights as they travel through their careers. Remember the point that was made at the start. The GP is doing the same thing on the day that they retire as they did on the day they started in practice. It is just that they are doing it much, much better.

What are the ethical issues that impact on your practice?

The General Medical Council (GMC) regulates doctors in the UK. They register doctors to practise in the UK and have the powers to issue a warning to a doctor, remove the doctor from the register, suspend or place conditions on a doctor's registration. The Medical Act 1983 provides the legal basis for everything that the GMC does.

The ethical base of doctoring is age-old and well entrenched. In general practice the needs of the patient are paramount. Confidentiality is supremely important. Many doctors will keep little more than cursory aides-memoires about the more sensitive matters that they discuss with their patient; many will decline to enter anything of this kind on a computer. These are issues that are becoming fraught in our current political climate. The most important principle is that the patient needs to know that the doctor can be trusted not to reveal anything to outsiders. This respect for patient confidentiality is an essential part of good care and applies to children and young people as well as to adults. Without the trust that confidentiality brings, children and young people might not seek medical care and advice, or they might not tell you, the doctor, all of the facts needed to provide good care. However, there are very rare circumstances in which it may be necessary to disclose information about a patient without their consent (GMC, 2007).

All doctors who are registered with the GMC are personally accountable for their professional practice and must always be prepared to justify their decisions and actions. The GMC's *Good Medical Practice* guidance (2006) sets out the principles and values on which this good professional practice is founded. These principles describe medical professionalism in action. The guidance is addressed to doctors, but you may find it interesting to read (see Further reading) as it is also intended to let the public know what they can expect from their doctors.

Working with people can be very demanding. How do you care for yourself?

Although general practitioners work in teams the nature of their work is very solitary. Stresses and difficulties can be shared with colleagues within the practice. Some GPs belong to peer support groups but this is unusual. In the end the GP is on their own and this can lead to pressures on their mental and physical health. Unfortunately GPs do not have a good record of handling this. Often they will self-medicate (a practice fraught with difficulties). In the *Good Medical Practice* guidance (2006) the GMC emphasises 'that doctors should not treat themselves and should be registered with a doctor to get independent medical advice about their own health'. Sometimes they will resort to alcohol and, very occasionally, to misuse of addictive drugs. One of the recommendations of the Shipman Inquiry (DoH, 2005) was that it should be made a criminal offence for doctors to self-prescribe controlled drugs, from their own or practice stock, except in an emergency.

The BMA (2007) cites international evidence that suggests that doctors are at a higher risk than the general population of developing stress-related problems, depression or suicide. Suicide rates among female NHS doctors have been shown to be twice that of the general female population, with rates for GPs being significantly higher than for doctors in hospital medicine. It is both a frightening and appalling fact that so many GPs kill themselves, yet little appears to be done, either by the profession or by society as a whole, to diminish these mortality rates.

How are your continuing professional development needs fulfilled and how do you ensure that your practice responds to current research?

GPs have a responsibility to ensure that their knowledge and skills are up to date and that they are familiar with relevant guidelines and developments. There has long been a requirement to take part in educational activities that maintain and further develop competence and performance. We must also keep up to date with, and adhere to, relevant laws and codes of practice.

So GPs' professional development needs are profuse, not only in understanding how they are working but in keeping abreast with all the different branches of medicine. Fortunately, there is no shortage of materials and methods. The Royal College of General Practitioners has, for more than two decades, developed a form of peer review of doctors and their practice. This is recognised as a route to Fellowship of the College and entails an in-depth look at all aspects of practice, both as an individual and as a member of a group.

How do you manage the conflicting demands of working with service users, colleagues and managers?

A number of different health care professionals work with the GP and the *Good Medical Practice* guidelines (2006) set out the expectations of the GMC with regard to the way in which all work together.

GPs are expected to provide primary care services to all the patients on their list. There can be no waiting list. All problems have to be addressed when they present. This is the primary concern of the doctor. However, today this primary concern is being challenged by a vast number of other agendas or targets (102 at the latest count) set up by the paymaster (government). Because achieving those 102 targets is tied to a doctor's remuneration it is inevitable that their attention will be focused on them rather than on patient need. When I go and see my doctor because I fear that my memory is going I do not want part of my valuable ten minutes to be taken up with measuring my blood pressure for the third time in two years, nor in having my blood taken to measure my cholesterol level, nor in being cross-questioned about how much exercise I take.

Key learning points

- A defining characteristic of general practice is its longitudinal nature.
- There are many antecedents to the consultation between patient and doctor.
- The GP brings to the consultation the skills of active listening, challenging, exploring and helping in the modification of the patient's story as well as recognising and treating disease.
- Between the two of them, patient and doctor work to create health.

REFLECTION ACTIVITIES

1. What do you think are the most important qualities of a GP?
2. Think about your own relationship with your GP. In what way is it a partnership?
3. Think about the last time that you visited your GP. Identify the interpersonal skills that were used.
4. Suicide rates for GPs are significantly higher than those for other doctors (BMA, 2007). Why do you think this is?

FURTHER READING

Balint, M. (1957) *The Doctor, His Patient and the Illness*. London: Pitman Medical; 2nd Ed. 1964; reprinted 1986. Edinburgh: Churchill Livingstone

Bendix, T. and Wright, H. (Eds) (1982) *The Anxious Patient*. Edinburgh: Churchill Livingstone

Brody, H. (2002) *Stories of Sickness* (2nd Ed.). Oxford: Oxford University Press

GMC (2006) *Good Medical Practice: The Duties of a Doctor Registered with the GMC*. Online at: **www.gmc-uk.org/guidance/good_medical_practice/duties_of_a_doctor.asp** (accessed 28 March 2008)

Glossary

Attending Showing another person that they have your full attention. This is achieved through body language and acknowledgement of feelings.

Cognitive behavioural therapy A type of talking therapy that focuses on changing both thinking and behaviour.

Congruence Being genuine or real.

Counselling A formal, confidential arrangement begun by the client in which a counsellor helps the client to explore their difficulties.

Counselling skills A range of communication skills that can be used by those in the helping professions to help service users.

Counter-transference Occurs when the subject of the transference responds as if they were the other person.

Empathy The ability to imagine what it must be like to be in someone else's situation.

Evidence-based practice Basing professional decisions on the best available research.

Experiential Knowledge based on experience in practice.

Humanistic A psychological approach that emphasises the human capacity for growth.

Immediacy The skill of using something that is happening in the present to help someone understand a situation or relationship.

Longitudinal Lengthwise or over a period of time.

Marginalised people or groups   People living on the edges of society such as homeless people, asylum seekers, etc.

Paraphrasing   The skill of identifying the meaning behind what someone says.

Pedagogy   The art of teaching.

Police staff   Non-sworn staff (previously known as civilians). Includes operational (police community support officers and scene of crime officers) as well as support and clerical staff.

Reflecting   Enabling another person to hear the words that they have spoken by repeating a word or phrase that they have used.

Reflection   Consideration or contemplation of a personal or professional issue.

Reflexive   An awareness of the influence of the professional identity, i.e. personality, beliefs, approach, on the casework relationship.

Respite care   Relief care to provide a carer with a break.

Summarising   Identifying the key points of what has been said.

Supervision   The formal relationship between a professional and colleague (usually more experienced or senior) for the purposes of gaining support and professional insight.

Therapeutic   Attempts to overcome illness.

Transference   Occurs when feelings, perceptions or expectations are projected onto another person.

Unconditional positive regard   An open approach in which individuals are viewed without prejudice or assumption.

Vulnerable adults   A technical term for the groups of adults traditionally identified in welfare law as being dependent and in need of welfare services such as, for example, adults with learning disabilities, those with physical disabilities, people with mental illness.

References

Adam, S.K. and Osborne, S. (2005) *Critical Care Nursing* (2nd Ed.). Oxford: Oxford University Press

Arthur, J., Davison, J. and Lewis, M. (2005) *Professional Values and Practice: Achieving the Standards for QTS.* London: RoutledgeFalmer

ATL, DfES, GMB, NAHT, NASUWT, NEOST, PAT, SHA, TGWU, UNISON, WAG (2003) *Raising Standards and Tackling Workload: A National Agreement.* Online at: **www.tda.gov.uk/upload/resources/na_standards_workload.pdf** (accessed 7 February 2008)

BACP (2007) *Ethical Framework for Good Practice in Counselling and Psychotherapy.* Online at: **www.bacp.co.uk/admin/structure/files/pdf/ethical_framework_web.pdf** (accessed 22 March 2008)

Balint, M. (1957) *The Doctor, His Patient and the Illness.* London: Pitman Medical (2nd Ed. 1964; reprinted 1986. Edinburgh: Churchill Livingstone)

Bartell, C. (2005) *Cultivating High Quality Teaching through Induction and Mentoring.* Thousand Oaks, CA: Corwin Press

BASW (2002) *Code of Ethics.* Online at: **www.basw.co.uk/Default.aspx?tabid=64uired** (accessed 18 March 2008)

Beauchamp, T. and Childress, J. (2001) *Principles of Biomedical Ethics* (5th Ed.). New York: Oxford University Press

Begat, I. and Severinsson, E. (2006) 'Reflection on how clinical nursing supervision enhances nurses' experience of well being related to their psychosocial work environment'. *Journal of Nursing Management* 14: 610–616

Berne, E. (1961) *Transactional Analysis in Psychotherapy.* New York: Grove Press

Berne, E. (1972) *What Do You Say After You Say Hello?* New York: Corgi Press

Biestek, P.P. (1957) *The Casework Relationship.* London: Allen & Unwin

BMA (2007) *Doctor's Health Matters.* Online at: **www.bma.org.uk/ap.nsffContent/doctorshealth~Doctorshealthintro7OpenDocument&Highlight=2,suicide,doctor** (accessed 28 May 2008)

Brody, H. (2002) *Stories of Sickness* (2nd Ed.). Oxford: Oxford University Press

Bubb, S. and Earley, P. (2004) *Managing Teacher Workload: Work–Life Balance and Wellbeing.* London: Paul Chapman

Burnard, P. (2006) *Counselling Skills for Health Professionals* (4th Ed.). Cheltenham: Nelson Thornes

Bush, K. (2001) 'Are you really listening to your patient?' *Registered Nurse*, 64(3): 35–7

Cambridge University Press (2008) *Cambridge Advanced Learners Dictionary*. Online at: **http://dictionary.cambridge.org/define. asp?key=80772&dict=CALD** (accessed 4 February 2008)

Canfield, J. and Hansen, V. (1996) *Chicken Soup for the Soul*. Deerfield Beach, FL: Health Communications

Centre for Evidence-based Social Services (2004) *Evidence-based Social Care*. Online at: **www.ripfa.org.uk/aboutus/archive/files/newsletters/ newsletter16/pdf** (accessed 21 June 2008)

Chapman, A. (n.d.) 'Beyond the Silence'. (Unpublished)

Chapman, C.M. (1983) 'The paradox of nursing'. *Journal of Advanced Nursing*, 8: 269–72

Clements, P. and Jones, J. (2006) *The Diversity Training Handbook: A Practical Guide to Understanding and Changing Attitudes* (2nd Ed.). London: Kogan Page

Cuthbert, S. and Quallington, J. (2008) *Values for Care Practice*. Exeter: Reflect Press

Dawes, M. *et al.* (2005) *Sicily Statement on Evidence-based Practice*. Online at: **www.biomedcentral.com/1472-6920/5/1** (accessed 21 July 2008)

DfES (2000) *Research into Teacher Effectiveness. A Model for Teacher Effectiveness*. Hay McBeal. Online at: **www.dfes.gov.uk/research/programmeofresearch/ projectinformation.cfm?projectid=12734&restultspage=1** (accessed 14 February 2008)

DfES (2005) *Primary National Strategy: Relationships in the Classroom*. Nottingham: TSO

DfES (2006) *The Common Assessment Framework for Children and Young People: Practitioners' Guide*. London: DfES

Dickinson, D.A., Hargie, O. and Morrow, N.C. (1989) *Communication Skills Training for Health Care Professionals*. London: Chapman & Hall.

Diggins, M. (2004) *Teaching and Learning Communication Skills in Social Work Education*. London: Social Care Institute for Excellence

DoH (1993) *Changing Childbirth: The Report of the Expert Maternity Group*. London: HMSO

DoH (2000) *No Secrets: Guidance on Developing and Implementing Multi-Agency Policies and Procedures to Protect Vulnerable Adults from Abuse*. Online at: **www.dh.gov.uk/en/Publicationsandstatistics/Publications/ PublicationsPolicyAndGuidance/DH_4008486** (accessed 22 May 2008)

DoH (2004a) *National Service Framework for Children, Young People and Maternity Services*. London: Department of Health/Department for Education and Skills

DoH (2004b) *The Ten Essential Shared Capabilities – A Framework for the Whole of the Mental Health Workforce*. London: Department of Health

DoH (2005) *The Shipman Inquiry*. Online at: **www.the-shipman-inquiry.org. uk/home.asp** (accessed 28 May 2008)

DoH (2008) *Social Work Careers Information*. Online at: **www.socialworkcareers. co.uk** (accessed 22 August 2008)

DoH/Partnerships for Children, Families and Maternity (2007) *Maternity*

Matters: Choice, Access and Continuity of Care in a Safe Service. London: Department of Health

Dohrenwend, A. (2002) 'Serving up the feedback sandwich'. *Family Practice Management*, 9 (10): 43–6

Dominelli, L. (2002) 'Anti-oppressive practice in context' in Adams, R., Dominelli, L. and Payne, M. (Eds) *Social Work: Themes, Issues and Critical Debates* (2nd Ed.). London: TSO

Donnelly, E. and Neville, L. (2008) *Communication and Interpersonal Skills.* Exeter: Reflect Press

Dowling, S., Barrett, S. and West, R. (1995) 'With nurse practitioners, who needs house officers?' *British Medical Journal*, 311: 309–13

Edwins, J. (2008) 'From a different planet', in Wickham, S. (Ed) *Midwifery: Best Practice*, Vol. 1. Hale: Books for Midwives Press

Egan, G. (1998) *The Skilled Helper.* Chichester: Wiley

Fish, F. and Coles, C. (2005) *Medical Education: Developing a Curriculum for Practice.* Maidenhead: McGraw-Hill International

Freud, S. (1894) 'The neuropsychosis of defence'. Reprinted (1953–1974) in *Standard Edition of the Complete Psychological Works of Sigmund Freud* (Trans. and Ed. J. Strachey), Vol. 3. London: Hogarth Press

Gardner, H. (1993) *Frames of Mind: The Theory of Multiple Intelligences* (2nd Ed.). London: Fontana Press

General Medical Council (2006) *Good Medical Practice: The Duties of a Doctor Registered with the GMC.* Online at: **www.gmc.uk.org/guidance/good_medical_practice/duties_of_a_doctor.asp** (accessed 28 March 2008)

General Medical Council (2007) *0–18 Years: Guidance for All Doctors.* Online at: **www.gmc-uk.org/guidance/archive/GMC_0-18.pdf** (accessed 28 May 2008)

General Teaching Council for England (2006a) *Statement of Professional Values and Practice for Teachers.* Birmingham: GTC Publications

General Teaching Council for England (2006b) *Using Research in Your School and Your Teaching.* Birmingham: GTC Publications

General Teaching Council for England (2007) *Making CPD Better. Bringing Together Research about CPD.* Birmingham: GTC Publications

George, J.B. (2001) *Nursing Theories – The Base for Professional Nursing Practice* (5th Ed.). Englewood Cliffs: Prentice Hall

Ginott, H. (1972) Cited in Rogers, B. (Ed.) (2004) *How to Manage Children's Challenging Behaviour.* London: Sage

Goleman, D. (1996) *Emotional Intelligence. Why It Can Matter More than IQ.* London: Bloomsbury

Gray, S.L. (2005) *An Enquiry into the Continuing Professional Development for Teachers.* Cambridge: University of Cambridge on behalf of the Esmée Fairbairn Foundation and Villiers Park Educational Trust

Hayes, J. (2002) *Interpersonal Skills at Work.* London: Routledge

Healthcare Commission (2007) *Annual Survey of NHS Staff.* Online at: **www.healthcarecommission.org.uk/newsandevents/pressreleases.cfm?widCall1=customWidgets.content_view_1&cit_id=6422** (accessed 8 May 2008)

Healy, K. (2005) *Social Work Theories in Context: Creating Frameworks for Practice*. Basingstoke: Palgrave Macmillan

Hendrick, J. (2000) *Law and Ethics in Nursing and Health Care*. Cheltenham: Stanley Thornes

Heron, J. (1990) *Helping the Client*. London: Sage

Hodnett, E.D., Lowe, N., Hannah, M.E. *et al.* (2002) 'Effectiveness of nurses as providers of birth labour support in North American Hospitals: a RCT'. *Journal of the American Medical Association*, 288: 1373–81

Holland, K. (2003) *Applying the Roper-Tierney Model in Practice*. London: Elsevier Health Services

Hook, P. and Vass, A. (2000) *Confident Classroom Leadership*. London: Fulton

Hopson, B. (1981) *Counselling and Helping in Psychology and Medicine*. London: Macmillan

Howe, D. (1987) *An Introduction to Social Work Theory*. Aldershot: Arena

Howe, D. (2008) *The Emotionally Intelligent Social Worker*. Basingstoke: Palgrave Macmillan

International Confederation of Midwives (2005) *Definition of the Midwife*. Online at: **www.internationalmidwives.org/Portals/5/Documentation/ICM%20Definition%20of%20the%20Midwife%202005.pdf** (accessed 6 August 2007)

Jones, P. (1998) *Holism: Making Sense of It All*. Online at: **www.p-jones.demon.co.uk/hcmholis.html** (accessed 8 May 2008)

Keogh, A. (2007) *PEACE Interviews*. Online at: **www.wikicrimeline.co.uk/index.php?title=PEACE_Interviews** (accessed 21 April 2008)

Kolb, D. (1984) *Experiential Learning: Experience as the Source of Learning and Development*. Englewood Cliffs, NJ: Prentice Hall

Lewis, G. (Ed.) (2004) *Why Mothers Die 2000–2002 – Report on Confidential Enquiries into Maternal Deaths in the United Kingdom*. London: RCOG

Lindon, J. and Lindon, L. (2000) *Mastering Counselling Skills*. Basingstoke: Palgrave

McHale, J. and Tingle, J. (2007) *Law and Nursing* (3rd Ed.). Oxford: Butterworth-Heinemann

McLeod, J. (2008) 'Embedded Counselling'. *Therapy Today*. 19(2): 4–7

McNally, R.J., Bryant, R.A. and Ehlers, A. (2003) 'Does Early Psychological Intervention Promote Recovery from Post Traumatic Stress?' *Psychological Science in the Public Interest*, 4(2): 45–79

Maslow, A. (1970) *Motivation and Personality* (3rd edn). New York: HarperCollins

Mearns, D. and Dryden, W. (1990) *Experiences of Counselling in Action*. London: Sage

Mental Health Nursing Association (1995) 'Clinical supervision'. *Mental Health Nursing*, (15)1. Online at: **www.amicus-mhna.org/guideclinsupervision.htm** (accessed 8 December 2008)

Milner-Bolotin, M. (2007) 'Teachers as actors'. *Physics Teacher*, 45(7): 459–61

Moon, J. (1999) *Reflection in Learning and Professional Development*. Abingdon: Routledge

Mulraney, S. (2001) 'Treating trauma'. *Police Review*, 2 March, pp. 23–4

Multiple Sclerosis Society (2007) *About MS*. Online at: **www.mssociety.org.uk/ about_ms/index.html About MS** (accessed 4 February 2008)

NAPWA (2007) V*alues, Principles and Moral Qualities for Police Welfare Advisers*. Online at: **www.policewelfare.co.uk/valuesandprincipals.htm** (accessed 22 March 2008)

National Union of Teachers (1999) *Tackling Stress*, NUT Health and Safety Briefing. Oneline at: **www.teachers.org.uk/resources/word/tackling_stress. doc** (accessed 14 March 2008)

National Union of Teachers (2007) *Tackling Stress – 2007 Update*, NUT Guidance to Divisions and Associations. Oneline at: **www.teachers.org.uk/ resources/word/TACKLING%20STRESS%20-%202007%20UPDATE_ PB.doc** (accessed 14 March 2008)

Neville, L. (2007) *The Personal Tutor's Handbook*. Basingstoke: Palgrave Macmillan

Nias, J. (1989) *Primary Teachers Talking: A Study of Teaching at Work*. London: Routledge

NICE (2003) *Management of Multiple Sclerosis in Primary and Secondary Care*. Online at: **www.nice.org.uk/nicemedia/pdf/cg008guidance.pdf** (accessed 24 March 2008)

Nursing and Midwifery Council (2004a) *Midwives Rules and Standards*. London: NMC

Nursing and Midwifery Council (2004b) *Protecting the Public through Professional Standards*. London: NMC

Nursing and Midwifery Council (2006a) *Standards for the Preparation and Practice of Supervisors of Midwives*. London: NMC

Nursing and Midwifery Council (2006b) *Clinical Supervision*. London: NMC

Nursing and Midwifery Council (2008a) *The Code: Standards of Conduct, Performance and Ethics for Nurses and Midwives*. London: NMC

Nursing and Midwifery Council (2008b) *Standards for Medicines Management*. London: NMC

Orem, D.E. (2001) *Nursing: Concepts of Practice* (6th Ed.). St Louis, MO: Mosby

Pairman, S. (2000) 'Women-centred midwifery: partnerships or professional friendships?', in Kirkham, M. (Ed.) *The Midwife–Mother Relationship*. Basingstoke: Palgrave Macmillan

Payne, M. (2005) *Modern Social Work Theory* (3rd Ed.). Basingstoke: Palgrave

Peplau, H.E. (1992) *Interpersonal Relations in Nursing*. London: Macmillan

Perrin Ouimet, K. and McGhee, J. (2001) *Ethics and Conflict*. Boston: Jones & Bartlett

Pickard, P. (2000) 'An inside job'. *Counselling News*, Summer, no. 25

Prosser, J. (1999) *School Culture*. London: Paul Chapman

Redmond, B. (2006) *Reflection in Action: Developing Reflective Practice in Health and Social Services*. Englewood Cliffs, NJ: Prentice Hall Health

Roberts, R., Trowell, T. and Golding, J. (2001) *Foundations of Health Psychology*. Basingstoke: Palgrave Macmillan

Rogers, C.R. (1959) 'A theory of therapy, personality, and interpersonal relationships as developed in the client-centered framework'. Reprinted in

Kirschenbaum, H. and Henderson, V. (Eds) (1989) *The Carl Rogers Reader*. Boston: Houghton Mifflin

Rogers, C. (1978) *Personal Power: Inner Strength and Its Revolutionary Impact*. London: Constable

Rogers, M.E. (1970) *An Introduction to the Theoretical Basis of Nursing*. Philadelphia: F.A. Davis

Roper, N., Logan, W.W. and Tierney, A.J. (1996) *The Elements of Nursing* (4th Ed.). Edinburgh: Churchill Livingstone

Roter, D.L., Hall, J.A. and Aoki, Y. (2002) 'Physician gender effects in medical communication: a meta-analytic review'. *Journal of the American Medical Association*, 288: 756–64. Online at: **www.bmj.com/cgi/content/short/336/7647/748#REF14** (accessed 5 April 2008)

Royal College of Psychiatrists (2003) *The Mental Health of Students in Higher Education*, Council Report CR112. London: Royal College of Psychiatrists

Seden, J. (2005) *Counselling Skills in Social Work Practice* (2nd Ed.). Maidenhead: Open University Press

Seedhouse, D. (1988) *Ethics: The Heart of Health Care*. Chichester: John Wiley & Sons

Seymour, L. and Grove, B. (2005) *Workplace Interventions for People with Common Mental Health Problems*. London: British Occupational Health Research Foundation

Snow, S. (2008) 'Personal health', in Edwins, J. (Ed.) *Community Midwifery Practice*. Oxford: Blackwell

Stokes, A. (2001) 'Settings' in Aldridge, S. and Rigby, S. (Eds) *Counselling Skills in Context*. London: Hodder & Stoughton

Teacher Support Network. (2007) *Worklife Balance*. Online at: **www.teachersupport.info** (accessed 16 February 2008)

Tennant, J. and Butler, S. (2007) Helping Women: the Use of Heron's Framework in Midwifery Practice. *British Journal of Midwifery*, 15(7): 425–428

Thompson, N. (2005) *Understanding Social Work: Preparing for Practice* (2nd Ed.). Maidenhead: Open University Press

Thompson, P. (2006) *People Problems*. Basingstoke: Palgrave Macmillan

Thorneycroft, G. (2006) *Shunned: Discrimination against People with Mental Illness*. Oxford: Oxford University Press

Training and Development Agency for Schools (2007a) *Reviewing Your School Policy for CPD*. London: TDA Publications

Training and Development Agency for Schools (2007b). *Effective Continuing Professional Development*. Online at: **www.tda.gov.uk/teachers/continuingprofessionaldevelopment/cpd_guidance/effective_cpd.aspx** (accessed 15 February 2008)

Wolsey, P. and Leach, L. (1997) 'Clinical supervision: a hornet's nest?', *Nursing Times*, 93: 24–6

World Health Organisation (2001) *Mental Health and Mental Illness in the UK*. Online at: **www.esrcsocietytoday.ac.uk/ESRCInfoCentre/facts/UK/index56.aspx?ComponentId=12917&SourcePageId=18133** (accessed 26 August 2008)

Index